THE

SIMPLE HEART CURE

Dr. Crandall's 90-Day Program to Stop and Reverse Heart Disease

THE

SIMPLE HEART CURE

Dr. Crandall's 90-Day Program to Stop and Reverse Heart Disease

Chauncey Crandall, M.D.

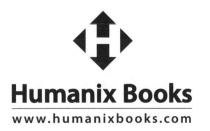

Humanix Books

www.humanixbooks.com

Humanix Books
The Simple Heart Cure

© 2013 Chauncey Crandall, M.D.
A Humanix Books publication

Humanix Books
P.O. Box 20989
West Palm Beach, FL 33416
www.humanixbooks.com
email: info@humanixbooks.com

Humanix Books is a division of Humanix Publishing LLC. Its trademark, consisting of the words "Humanix Books" is registered in the U.S. Patent and Trademark Office and in other countries.

Disclaimer: The information presented in this book is not specific medical advice for any individual and should not substitute medical advice from a health professional. If you have (or think you may have) a heart problem or heart disease, speak to your doctor or a health professional immediately about your risk and possible treatments. Do not engage in any care of treatment without consulting a medical professional.

Printed in the United States of America

ISBN (Hardcover) 978-1-63006-007-7
ISBN (E-Book) 978-1-63006-008-1

LCCN 2013944532

To my wife, Deborah, my sons Christian and Chad,
and for the patients the Lord has entrusted to my care.
All to the glory of God.

TABLE OF CONTENTS

Part Three: Fix It!

Your First Step to Be Heart Disease Free

W elcome to *The Simple Heart Cure: Dr. Crandall's 90-Day Program to Stop and Reverse Heart Disease*. Congratulations on taking the initiative to reach out for information that will help you to guard your heart's health and live the life that God intended. I hope you'll find this book an invaluable resource.

No doubt you are reading this book because you have concerns. Maybe you've already had a heart attack. Or you've been suffering from angina and are wondering about new and improved treatments. You may be overweight, plagued by a smoking habit, or your doctor has told you that your cholesterol counts are through the roof. It's natural to worry.

Heart disease is the No. 1 killer in America, not only for men but women as well. In fact, heart disease kills more women every year than all cancers combined — including breast cancer. Nearly a third of all deaths are from heart disease.

It's not as if there's not enough information out there. In fact, there's almost too much: Internet sites, shelves upon shelves of books, pamphlets, newsletters, television shows, and advertisements for every treatment imaginable.

Understandably, many people suffer from information overload. We'd like just to trust our doctors, but they have waiting rooms crammed full of patients. Too often, the easiest thing to do is reach for the prescription pad, rather than teaching and leading patients to better health.

My Journey From Tribal Life to Modern Doctor

Who am I? I'm a Yale Medical School-trained, board-certified, interventional cardiologist (F.A.C.C., F.C.C.P.). I practice in Palm Beach,

Fla., and many of America's most powerful and wealthy people, including many billionaires, are among my patients. In fact, people fly in from all over America and from abroad to see me. Of course, I take care of many people of modest means but I am especially drawn to the care of the elderly and the poor.

From an early age, I was interested in medicine, but during my college and early graduate years, I also was fascinated by anthropology — the study of human beings and their cultures. This interest endures and has enabled me to see things other Western physicians often cannot see.

As an undergraduate, I traveled to the West African nation of Togo to study the Kabre tribe. The Kabre live on a diet of cereals, fruits, and vegetables, consuming meat only on feasting occasions. Heart disease is almost unknown among them. I became interested in specializing in cardiology during my medical training, so I volunteered to assist in cutting-edge research. This added to the workload, but it was well worth it.

From 1989 to 1993, I was on the clinical research faculty at the Medical College of Virginia in Richmond, Va. There, I ran the heart transplant program. This involved assessing every transplant candidate's eligibility.

This was truly "holistic" medicine, in the sense that everything had to be considered — the patient's prior behavior, the presence or absence of other health conditions, the ability of his family to support his recovery — before a candidate received the green light for (or was denied) a new heart.

The Wake-Up Call: My Own Heart Battle

Then I had the most enlightening day in my lifelong study of heart disease: I became a patient.

In 2002, I was returning from a speaking engagement on Long Island. When I arrived at the airport in New York, I pulled my suitcase out of the car and felt a sharp pain in my shoulder.

But I was only 48, not a diabetic, I don't smoke, and I have no family history of heart disease. It simply didn't occur to me then that it might be my heart. I boarded the plane, and the pain went away. When I arrived in Palm Beach, I picked up my bag, and the pain in my shoulder came back, now with a little pressure in my chest. But I was fine by the time I arrived home.

I didn't want to tell my wife, Deborah. I kept going through possible diagnoses in my head, trying to convince myself that it couldn't be heart disease.

My wife runs in the morning. I thought I'd walk along behind her, but I couldn't even make it to the end of the driveway without severe pain. I sat on the entryway steps and waited until she returned.

It was hard to admit, but I finally said it out loud: "Deborah, you have to take me to the hospital. I've got a heart problem." By the time the medical team had me on the table, I was in severe pain.

My whole heart was crying out for blood, and it couldn't get any — my left anterior descending (LAD) coronary artery was 99 percent blocked! I had an emergency angioplasty and received two stents.

I learned from this episode that if I wanted to continue making a significant contribution to this world, I had to take care of my health. I had to get serious about exercise, stay on a restricted diet, get a periodic stress test, and pray for the healing of my body, for my own and my family's sake. That's why I'm so glad you are reading this book. Consider it a "virtual visit" with one of your doctors. (It should not, however, be considered a substitute for consulting with your personal physician. I would never advise that.)

I believe strongly that if you read this book and use the Three Keys — Learn It, Treat It, and Reverse It — you will focus on the changes you need to make and achieve victory over heart disease.

Let's get started!

INTRODUCTION

I dread the emergency calls that send me flying down the hospital corridor when patients are brought to the hospital in cardiac arrest. I know the news is not likely to be good; many times, patients brought into the hospital this late after suffering a heart attack don't make it. But nothing prepared me for the shock of seeing my good friend Jack lying there on the gurney.

Earlier that day Jack had started suffering discomfort after one of his customary indulgent meals, which he'd topped off with a cigar. He ignored the growing discomfort in his shoulder, brushed aside his wife's growing concern, as he grew pale and sweaty. But he waited four hours, until he was writhing in pain, his face contorted in agony, before he finally gave in to her pleas to call an ambulance. But it was too late.

Although oxygen was started as the ambulance screamed its way to the hospital, by the time Jack arrived there, he was gone. His daughter had cried out for me to save him, but there was nothing I could do. A sense of helplessness overwhelmed me.

This is the true story of a heart attack. Jack was only 54 years old. He was a hard worker, and had reached the pinnacle of his career, working for a world-famous luxury brand you'd recognize in an instant. He had a beautiful wife who loved him and two grown children upon whom he doted. They adored him right back. He was a man whom many people would have envied, had he not been such a nice guy. Instead, he was widely regarded as a pillar of our community, a distinction he had earned.

But Jack was overweight, and, because of that, he was saddled with all the health complications that come along with it: diabetes, high cholesterol and also high blood pressure. These comprise the constellation of conditions known as "metabolic syndrome," which drastically drives up heart attack risk.

Jack had come to me years before with complaints that turned out to be heart disease. I prescribed medications, along with diet and exercise. He took the medications but ignored the rest. His job called for him to wine and dine clients, which he did with gusto. His wife was powerless to help. I even called upon his secretary, who made his restaurant reservations (he often took clients to steakhouses for expense account meals), but all to no avail.

This went on, while he gained weight, and my sense of dread grew. And then, suddenly, just like that, he was gone. It's been a year now since he died on that horrible night, but each day, when I walk past where he worked, I feel that deep, sharp pain that comes from loss. If only Jack had paid heed, and made some simple changes in his life, we'd be standing in his office today, laughing and talking the way we once did. I would have done anything to stop the tragedy that unfolded, but he simply refused to listen to me. I miss him deeply.

My decision to write this book comes from that wellspring of loss, futility and needless death, the plight that befalls so many families whose loved ones are taken from them too soon.

With today's technology, if you get to the hospital in time, many heart attack victims can be saved. *The harsh fact, though, is that only 7 percent of the people who suffer cardiac arrest outside of a hospital can be saved.* Not only that, but about one-third of heart attack victims die without even experiencing symptoms; they succumb to a so-called "silent" heart attack.

But this doesn't have to happen to you. Every day, I see patients who have become victorious over heart disease. They tell me that they feel healthier, and happier than they did even before their heart attack. This doesn't surprise me at all; before their heart attack, they were sick, and just ticking time bombs. After they follow *The Simple Heart Cure* plan, they feel reborn.

Don't wait to have that first heart attack to transform your life. It could be too late.

Before you get any further into this book, I want you to go to the computer and go to *SimpleHeart411.com*. Once you're there, complete the 19 questions and you'll learn not only what your risk of heart disease is, but also the areas that you must change in order to save your life.

Really, don't wait — I tailored this book with this important first step in mind. This is the very first step you must take to save your heart.

After all, when you embark on any challenge, you need to know your starting point. Even when you start out to map a trip, you must know your starting point. Well, it is no different with the health of your heart.

Too often, people neglect to evaluate their risk factors, but how do you know what you need to change unless you do so? That's why I created the Simple Heart Test.

This was the easiest, quickest way I could think of that will give you an appraisal of where you stand, and what you must change to avoid that heart attack, the one that could be fatal, and take you away from your family.

So don't hesitate — just go to *SimpleHeart411.com* and answer the quick 19 questions. You'll receive an assessment back by email. Keep that alongside you, as you go through this book. And remember, as you go through this book, I'll be there every step of the way, to offer you guidance, tips, and to cheer you on!

So do it right now, and know that you're taking the first step to protect your heart, so you don't become a heart attack statistic like my friend Jack. Go to *SimpleHeart411.com* to assess your risk for heart attack in just minutes. It may save your life.

PART ONE

Learn It!

CHAPTER 1

The No. 1 Cause of Heart Disease – It's Hidden and Deadly

Here's a shocking statistic: 75 percent of all deaths from heart disease have a single cause that develops undetected over decades with no symptoms at all. The condition is atherosclerosis, commonly referred to as "hardening of the arteries."

Even people who appear healthy can be struck down by a sudden, fatal heart attack due to atherosclerosis. In June 2008, popular newsman Tim Russert was busy preparing for his show *Meet the Press* when he collapsed and died. His personal physician later issued a statement saying that Russert had "coronary artery disease that resulted in hard ening of his coronary arteries."

Six years earlier, the same thing happened to St. Louis Cardinals pitcher Darryl Kile. At age 33, Kile died in his sleep of a heart attack. This was a man in great physical shape. But two of Kile's coronary arteries were 90 percent blocked, even though he had no outward symptoms.

Hardening of the arteries develops over many years, often starting in childhood. Even very young children can develop fatty streaks and deposits in the lining of the arteries. One study found that 1 out of every 6 teenagers already has lesions, or damaged areas, in their arteries.

But this progressive condition has become an epidemic in the last 100 years. In 1900, coronary heart disease wasn't even in the top 10 causes of death in the United States. Now it affects half of all Americans and claims 500,000 lives each year.

How did we get to this point?

The Inflammatory Response

The arteries carry oxygenated blood from the heart and lungs to other parts of the body, feeding the organs with oxygen and other nutrients dissolved in the blood. When your arteries are healthy, they are smooth and elastic, allowing blood to flow freely.

But when fatty deposits start building up inside the arteries, the blood vessels narrow. This buildup is called plaque and it reduces the blood supply that an artery can process. The plaque also irritates the arterial wall and results in calcification, or "hardening" of the tissue.

The artery wall responds to irritation the same way skin does: It becomes inflamed. This is a good thing when you scrape your knee, because the redness, swelling, and warmth of inflammation keeps bacteria out of the wound, and increased blood supply brings extra white blood cells to begin the healing process.

The same thing happens when the inside of an artery is irritated and the body makes a "patch" over the irritation with cholesterol. However, in the limited space of the artery, that patch acts like a speed bump. When this happens repeatedly, arteries become riddled with lesions. They lose their elasticity and become narrow, and the heart has to work harder to push blood through — so your blood pressure goes up.

Worse yet, that patched area may grow, or a piece of the patch can break off and flow down the bloodstream until it reaches a smaller vessel and becomes a blockage. The artery might even rupture at a weak spot.

Understanding inflammation is important because it is the trigger that sets off artery damage. It also sustains the hardening effect. So what are the causes of inflammation in an artery?

The No. 1 source of inflammation in the body is a bad diet. That explains why hardening of the arteries has become an epidemic only in the last 100 years: Our diet has changed dramatically in that time.

For the great majority of human history, we were hunter-gatherers. That meant the human diet consisted of only what could be caught or harvested. The food supply varied from week to week and from season to season. There were times of plenty and times of need. The body had to store extra calories as fat to get through those lean times.

Today, we live a life of constant plenty. Everyone has a kitchen full of food all the time, and long before supplies get low, we drive to the supermarket for more.

And what do we buy when we get there? Refined foods that are convenient to store and eat, all of which are stocked with sugar, salt, and fat to make them taste good. Such foods are also high in omega-6 fats that promote inflammation. The body is forced to store all those excess calories as fat.

That's what it's supposed to do . . . but the lean times never come. The result? Lots of belly fat.

When you have a large, protruding belly, it means that you have what is known as visceral fat, which consists of fat deposits around your organs. That causes high risk for heart disease and hardening of the arteries.

Belly fat is dangerous because it releases what I call "inflammation mediators" into the bloodstream. These are chemicals that cause inflammation in the arteries, leading to artery damage. All the time you are maintaining belly fat, these mediators are circulating in your system and damaging your arteries.

When I travel to Third World countries on medical relief and mission trips, I rarely see people with belly fat. If there is a fat person, it's usually the richest person in the village because they are the only ones who can afford to overeat. And they are the ones with modern diseases like hardening of the arteries.

Symptoms of 'Global Devastation'

Hardening of the arteries doesn't just involve the heart. I call it "global devastation" of the body because the arteries go to all the vital organs, and when hardening sets in, any of those organs can be affected.

When the arteries to the heart are affected, the result can be:
- Angina (chest pain)
- Shortness of breath, sweating, and anxiety
- Abnormal heartbeat
- Congestive heart failure
- Heart attack

When the arteries to the brain are affected, the result can be:
- Numbness or weakness
- Loss of speech or difficulty swallowing
- Warning stroke, or TIA (transient ischemic attack)
- Full-fledged stroke that causes death of brain tissue
- Dementia and Alzheimer's disease

When the arteries to the extremities are affected, the result can be:
- Severe leg pain (claudication)
- Wounds that won't heal

Hardening of the arteries can also affect the eyes or the kidneys, or cause erectile dysfunction in men.

There are a number of medical exams your doctor can perform to measure your risk of heart disease due to hardening of the arteries. But first, here is a test you can do in the privacy of your own home that is very revealing. It's called the "waist-to-hip ratio."

This simple test — which requires nothing but a tape measure and a calculator — has proven to be a better predictor of heart disease than body mass index (BMI).

Here's what you do:

1. Measure the thinnest part of your waist
2. Measure the widest part of your hips
3. Divide the first measurement by the second one.

This is your waist-to-hip ratio.

Let's say your waist is 36" and your hips are 47"; 36 divided by 47 equals 0.765. A healthy ratio for women is anything less than 0.8. For men, it's less than 0.9.

If your ratio is higher than that, it probably means you have excess belly fat. Studies show that people with excess belly fat have more plaque in their arteries, putting them at greater risk for heart disease.

Your doctor may also want to do blood work to check your cholesterol and triglyceride levels. I like to see total cholesterol under 150 with HDL greater than 45 and LDL less than 70. Triglyceride count should be less than 150.

An electrocardiogram (EKG) looks at how electrical current travels through the heart. A resting EKG tells the rate and regularity of the heartbeat. But be warned: Electrical currents in the heart can be completely normal even when someone has severely blocked arteries.

A stress EKG is conducted while the patient exercises on a treadmill or stationary bike. Someone with arteriosclerosis will usually show evidence of decreased blood supply to the heart during exercise.

If any of these noninvasive tests indicate probability of atherosclerosis, an angiogram can be done. In this test, special dye is injected into the arteries, and X-rays track the dye as it travels through the body. This test is the gold standard for determining how advanced hardening of the arteries has become.

Lifestyle Change Is the First Step

The goal in treating arteriosclerosis is to restore as much blood flow as possible. If you already have advanced hardening of the arteries, the first line of defense is to get your blood pressure, blood sugar, and cholesterol under control — with medication if necessary. The next step is to control your risk factors by getting to the source of the problem. That means lifestyle changes.

You hear this all the time: Control your weight and get regular exercise. It's not new information, but it's vitally important because 85 percent of heart disease comes from lifestyle. Too much processed food and too many sedentary habits are the recipe for hardening of the arteries and heart disease.

If you're carrying extra belly fat, you have inflammatory mediators circulating in your system all the time; over the years, these do a lot of damage to the arteries. The best diet you can eat is lots of fresh produce, less eggs and red meat, and modest portions of fish and poultry.

One popular anti-inflammatory diet is called the Mediterranean diet because it emulates the traditional diet of southern Italy, Greece, and other countries around the Mediterranean Sea. It includes olive oil and nuts (in moderation) for monounsaturated fat. Fresh, cold-water fish high in omega-3 fats are a staple. These types of fats actually help reduce inflammation in the body — as long as you don't overdo it.

The American Heart Association's Lyon Diet Heart Study was conducted to test the effectiveness of the Mediterranean diet. The study followed 600 patients who had survived a first heart attack; half were given a Mediterranean-style diet (replacing butter and cream with a margarine high in omega-3 fatty acid); the other half followed a typical American diet.

After a year, the Mediterranean diet group was doing so much better than the control group that the study was stopped so everyone could have the opportunity to change their diet. In a follow up almost four years after the study started, patients following the Mediterranean-style diet had a 50 to 70 percent lower risk of recurrent heart disease. That's a significant improvement based on diet alone.

I also recommend the **South Beach diet** and the **Dean Ornish diet**. Both easy to find at your local bookstore. Women should keep their daily calorie count at around 1,500; men around 1,800.

Other Lifestyle Choices

We all know that there is no safe amount of smoking. Tobacco smoke damages the arteries and causes them to narrow. People who smoke a pack of cigarettes a day have twice the risk of heart attack as non-smokers. But the good news is that your risk of heart attack decreases in as little as 24 hours after quitting smoking. After one year, risk of heart disease is only half that of a current smoker, according to research conducted by the Cleveland Clinic.

Exercise helps keep arteries elastic, even in older people. That's why I tell my patients to get an hour of exercise a day at least five days a week. It keeps the blood flowing and reduces blood pressure. It also reduces inflammation and stress.

Stress is another major factor in arteriosclerosis. Under stress, your body releases the hormones adrenaline and cortisol, which prepare the body for "fight or flight." The heart speeds up, blood vessels constrict, and clotting factors are activated in case of possible injury. Your body is ready for an emergency.

Chronic stress, however, induces the same situation even when there isn't an emergency. Having your system "on alert" all the time creates inflammation and makes the arteries less flexible.

Experiments have shown that arteries become more elastic in response to physical stress (such as a bicycle exercise test) and less elastic under psychological stress (such as public speaking). In a study of patients with coronary artery disease, those whose blood pressure increased during a public speaking test were more likely to die within three years. According to a study published in the Harvard Mental Health Letter, those who developed chest pain during public speaking were three times more likely to suffer a cardiac event in the next five years.

All of us suffer stress from one source or another. That's just a fact of life. What is important is how you handle it. I advise my patients to cultivate family closeness as well as strong faith. Keeping our souls nourished is healing for the arteries and the heart.

Studies have shown that people without a strong network of friends or family are at much greater risk of heart disease. Why does this happen? Lonely people have higher levels of cortisol and inflammation. Loneliness has also been shown to make it harder for blood to move through the arteries, which raises blood pressure.

The interesting thing is that loneliness is a "perceived" emotion. Some people don't have a lot of social interaction but don't feel lonely because they need a lot of "me" time. Others have people around them all the time, but still don't feel connected. The connection is what is important.

This fact was illustrated in a study that consisted of interviews with nearly 1,300 patients who were scheduled to have coronary artery by-pass surgery. They were asked to respond "yes" or "no" to 38 statements regarding their mental and physical health, such as: "Things are getting me down," "I'm feeling on edge," and "I'm in constant pain."

Later, researchers compared the responses to the mortality rates of the patients (after controlling for risk factors such as age and smoking). It turned out that only one of the 38 statements — "I feel lonely" — was associated with mortality in both the short and long term.

Whether you have just a few close friends or a large family, the important thing is feeling connected. Talking with your spouse or a close friend is a powerful stress-reducer.

Hardening of the arteries is the underlying cause of most heart disease, which is the leading cause of death in the United States. The primary factors behind hardening of the arteries are diet and lifestyle. That's why it takes decades to develop.

So whether you already have arteriosclerosis or you just want to be sure that it never gets out of hand, pay attention to the lifestyle choices you make. It affects everyone to some degree, and results in heart disease in fully half of the population.

For some people, symptoms gradually develop as arteries become blocked and hardened. For others — like Tim Russert and Darryl Kile — the first symptom is a fatal heart attack.

Either way, controlling hardening of the arteries is the key to a healthy heart. And, as always, prevention is the best cure.

CHAPTER 2

A Ticking Time Bomb

Hall of Fame basketball player Jerry West always felt as if he had a "ticking time bomb" in his chest. During his 14-year career with the National Basketball Association's Los Angeles Lakers, he chalked the feeling up to being a highly competitive player in a physically demanding profession.

But the anxiety and sleeplessness that nagged him during his playing days didn't let up when he retired from basketball.

It was a long time before West discovered that the time bomb was atrial fibrillation — a condition in which the upper chambers of the heart (the atria) beat uncontrollably and out of coordination with the lower chambers (the ventricles). He had access to excellent medical care, yet his condition went undiagnosed for 30 years. In fact, he had been suffering from atrial fibrillation for most of his life.

An irregular heartbeat — also called a cardiac arrhythmia — is one of the most common things that can happen to the heart with age. I see it every day in my cardiology practice. Patients complain of their heart "pounding," "fluttering," or skipping beats. They often feel dizzy or short of breath.

The heart is basically a large electrical system. When this system is working correctly, you don't feel your heartbeat.

An irregular heartbeat occurs when the electrical system misfires. This misfiring most often is a result of simple wear and tear. Cardiac arrhythmias cause more than half a million people to be admitted to the hospital each year.

This electrical system — also called the cardiac conduction system — consists of three parts:

1. The sinoatrial (S-A) node, in the upper right chamber of the heart, is a natural pacemaker with special cells that create the electrical impulses that make your heart beat. The S-A node is the initiator of heartbeats. It keeps the heart firing in a consistent rhythm.

2. The atrialventricular (A-V) node is in the center of the heart, at the junction of the four chambers. It picks up the electric signals from the S-A node and passes them to the lower part of the heart.

3. The His-Purkinje system is a bundle of fibers that carries electricity through the lower chambers of the heart (the ventricles) and causes those chambers to contract to pump blood to the rest of the body.

The S-A node normally generates about 60 to 80 signals per minute, which determines your heart rate. In a healthy heart, the electric impulses travel through the three parts of the conduction system in a coordinated way, creating what is called a sinus rhythm.

This sinus rhythm speeds up when you exert yourself and slows down when you are asleep. But as long as the rhythm remains even, it is normal.

When the heart beats out of rhythm, it's not normal. What's more, it can be dangerous — the blood supply may be disrupted, and the tissues that rely on that blood for nourishment can be damaged.

Anyone can develop a cardiac arrhythmia at any age, but the condition is most common in people older than 65. As in the case of Jerry West, arrhythmias can go unnoticed for a long time. On the other hand, they may cause symptoms, such as chest pain, palpitations, weakness, dizziness, fainting, or even unexplained anxiety.

Most arrhythmias are labeled by the area of the heart where they occur: Atrial arrhythmias happen in the upper chambers of the heart, the atria; ventricular arrhythmias originate in the lower chambers of the heart, the ventricles. Cardiac arrhythmias are also classified by whether the heart beats too quickly (tachycardia) or too slowly (bradycardia).

Some arrhythmias are more serious than others, and each affects the body differently. First, I'll tell you about the risk factors and treatments for each type of arrhythmia. Later, I'll explain what you can do to minimize your risk of cardiac arrhythmia.

Treating Atrial Arrhythmias

There are two types of tachycardias that occur in the upper chambers of the heart, the atria:

1. An atrial flutter (AFL) is a fast, even heartbeat of about 250 to 350 beats per minute. This is a significant increase from the 60 to 80 beats per minute in a heart that is functioning correctly.

2. Atrial fibrillation (AFib) is even faster, with rates varying between 300 and 600 beats per minute. At this rate, the fibrillating chamber ceases to pump efficiently. Rather, it is quivering, and some blood is actually left behind in the chamber. That pooled blood can clot and increase the risk of stroke. People with chronic AFib are five times more likely to have a stroke than those with a normal heart beat.

But AFLs and AFibs don't always present the same symptoms. Some people experience mild fluttering in the chest or neck, while others complain of "pounding" that feels like a runaway train. Many people can feel dizzy or faint or short of breath because the heart is not pumping blood efficiently.

A number of things can cause atrial arrhythmias, including:

- Too vigorous exercise
- Stress
- Stimulants such as caffeine and nicotine
- Alcohol consumption
- Medications such as cough and cold medicines, decongestants, and asthma inhalers
- Underlying heart disease such as, high blood pressure and heart valve disorders
- Chronic lung disease such as asthma or emphysema
- Diabetes
- Thyroid disease
- Overheating of the body

Arrhythmias can be diagnosed with an electrocardiogram (EKG), a painless test in which electrode patches are attached to the chest to measure how the electrical signals are passing through your heart. A doctor can tell from the wave patterns what kind of rhythm your heart has.

If a physician suspects there could be an arrhythmia that might not show up during an EKG, you may need to wear a Holter monitor, a device that can record your heartbeat for 24 hours at home. Another option is to take a stress test to see whether exercise is triggering arrhythmias.

Treatment of atrial arrhythmias is varied. For mild cases, you may be able to simply avoid what is causing them.

I had one patient who experienced atrial fibrillation only after going out for a nice dinner. It turned out that alcohol was causing the arrhythmia. She and her husband and friends would have a cocktail or two before dinner, then a bottle of wine with the meal. Afterwards, her pulse was rapid and she felt fluttering in her chest. This is typical of alcohol-induced arrhythmias (often called "Holiday Heart Syndrome"). Avoiding alcohol solved her problem without further treatment.

Obviously, if you realize that caffeine, nicotine, or a decongestant makes your heart beat abnormally, then you should stay away from those things.

In more serious cases, your doctor may prescribe an anti-arrhythmic drug to help control your heart rate. You probably also will be prescribed an anti-coagulant (blood thinner) to reduce the risk of blood clots and stroke.

Ventricular Arrhythmias

There are also two types of ventricular (lower chamber) arrhythmias, both of which are deadly and require immediate medical attention:

1. **Ventricular tachycardia (VT)** is a very fast heart rhythm that acts like an electrical short circuit racing around in a circle at 150 to 250 beats per minute. Two things happen: One, the heart races and pumps less blood; two, there is not enough time for the heart chamber to fill with blood between beats. That interrupts blood flow to the point that the brain and the body do not get enough blood and oxygen.

2. **Ventricular Fibrillation (VFib)** causes the heart to beat in a very fast, chaotic way, sometimes reaching over 300 beats per minute. With this condition, the lower chamber quivers rather than pumps, so very little blood gets to the rest of the body. A person can become unconscious and die within minutes. Treatment with electric shock from a defibrillator must be done immediately to correct the rhythm.

If you experience VT, you may feel as if your heart is skipping beats. As the heartbeat gets faster, you may become dizzy, have blind spots, and even black out.

Ventricular arrhythmias can be challenging to diagnose and treat because they are very unpredictable. They might show up on an EKG. But sometimes they don't, and more invasive testing may be required.

To evaluate the electrical activity of the heart accurately, a doctor can perform an electrophysiology (EP) test, in which catheters are inserted through the groin and up to the heart while the patient is sedated but conscious. It gives a much clearer picture of heart activity than an EKG.

Because any episode of ventricular arrhythmia is a life-threatening event, it must be followed up with a thorough examination for underlying heart disease. Such episodes often occur to people who have sustained damage from a heart attack or cardiac surgery, or in those who have an inherited genetic heart disease.

In severe cases, a device called an implantable cardioverter defibrillator (ICD) can be implanted in the heart. It can be programmed to detect abnormal heart rhythms and not only deliver a shock to correct a VT or VFib but also record what happened. A physician then can analyze the data and adjust the settings on the device, if necessary.

Bradycardia: The Heart Beating Too Slow

Bradycardia is a condition in which the heart beats too slowly — usually less than 60 beats per minute. At that rate, the heart doesn't contract enough to supply adequate blood and oxygen to the body.

Naturally, if your heart is not pumping enough blood, you are going to feel tired, especially when you try to exert yourself. Symptoms include fatigue, dizziness and shortness of breath. A doctor can diagnose it with an ECG.

Bradycardia, which affects about 600,000 people a year, is most common in elderly people. But elderly people often think they are tired because they are getting older. If the symptoms develop gradually, which often is the case with bradycardia, people may not even realize they have a heart problem.

Everyone needs to understand: It's not normal to be too tired to get out of your chair! One patient of mine got exhausted just walking to the mailbox and back. If such things are happening, it's time to see a doctor and find out whether your heart needs to pick up the beat.

The most common treatment of bradycardia is to implant a pace-maker. This small device uses low-energy electrical pulses to help the heart beat at a normal rate. It can work wonders in helping a person resume a normal, active lifestyle.

Healthy Habits Equal Healthy Hearts

Unfortunately, when the heart's electrical system goes haywire, there is no one easy cure for the resulting arrhythmia. The key is to keep your heart healthy with lifestyle choices. The body has a remarkable ability to respond to healthy habits, so it is never too late to develop them.

What can you do to reduce the risk of developing heart arrhythmias with age? First of all, be aware of your heart health. If you notice that certain activities seem to upset the rhythm of your heart, then it is best to avoid them.

You also should educate yourself about common substances that can cause arrhythmias. For instance caffeine, nicotine, and alcohol are all known to disrupt the heart's rhythm. Many people find that their arrhythmia will stop completely if they just avoid coffee, tea, chocolate, soft drinks, and alcohol.

It's also important to avoid stress and anxiety. I talk a lot about the effects of stress on the heart because I see it every day in my practice. Stress is a silent destroyer, and learning to manage it is one of the best things you can do for your heart.

Sometimes, a good diet is just not enough to maintain a healthy heart. And if your diet is not so good, then you will need to take a good multivitamin at the very least. Take one every day just to ensure that you are getting the minimum nutrients you need.

Fish oil is the most concentrated source of the omega-3 fatty acids eicosapentaenoic acid (EPA) and docosapentaenoic acid (DHA). One study of more than 11,000 people taking omega-3 as a supplement showed a 45 percent reduction in sudden cardiac death. This reduction was seen even in patients already taking aspirin and statins for heart disease.

Fish oil helps stabilize the electrical activity of the heart muscle. The recommended dose is 2 grams per day of a supplement that contains both EPA and DHA. (Consult your doctor if you take a blood thinner, as fish oil may increase its effect.)

Magnesium can also help stabilize the heart's electrical system. Studies have shown that arrhythmias are more likely to occur when blood levels of magnesium are low. People with congestive heart failure are especially susceptible to arrhythmias when magnesium is low.

A diet high in processed foods is deficient in magnesium. Soft drinks and bottled water are devoid of magnesium. Anyone on diuretics probably will have low magnesium.

Magnesium supplements are safe and inexpensive, though they may cause diarrhea in doses of more than 250 mg. For that reason, it is best to take magnesium in divided doses throughout the day. The total daily dose is 300 to 500 mg.

Because arrhythmias so often are caused or aggravated by underlying heart disease, the same guidelines that apply to managing heart disease can be applied to managing arrhythmias. I always recommend that patients eat a plant-based diet such as the Mediterranean diet or stick to the Dean Ornish Program.

There's absolutely no substitute for the fiber and nutrition God puts into fresh fruits and vegetables. Eating well and staying at a healthy weight will help your heart to function normally.

Regular exercise keeps your heart in good shape, but you should be modest about sports if you have an arrhythmia. Competitive activities may be too much for someone with an abnormal heart rhythm. Consult your physician if you want to increase your activity to that level.

As I said, I see arrhythmias every day. They are part of the aging of the electrical system of the heart — and they will continue to become more common in the U.S., where the average life expectancy is 77.

By contrast, I don't see very many arrhythmias when I travel to Third World countries, where life expectancy is a mere 49. People in those countries simply don't live long enough to develop many of the heart problems we see here.

Arrhythmias may be more common with age, but they are not inevitable. Practicing a healthy lifestyle will go a long way toward preventing both heart disease and arrhythmias.

If you follow the advice I give in these pages and pay attention to the advice of your physician, you can avoid the ticking time bomb of cardiac arrhythmias.

To better understand if you are at risk for cardiac arrhythmia, go to *www.simpleheart411.com* and take my simple heart test now.

CHAPTER 3

7 Hidden Risk Factors

I told you earlier about my own heart experience. I had arrived at LaGuardia Airport and pulled my suitcase out of the car when I felt a sharp pain in my shoulder and later my chest.

I tried to ignore it. In my mind, I went through the major risk factors for heart disease: high blood pressure, diabetes, smoking, high cholesterol.

I had none of those major risk factors, and so I was convinced that the pain I was feeling was not the signal of an impending heart attack.

But the next day, it was even worse. I finally went to the hospital, where tests showed that I had a buildup of plaque in the blood vessels of the heart called atherosclerosis. An emergency angioplasty and stent fixed me up, but I knew that, if I didn't find out what had caused my heart disease and address it, I'd be back in the emergency room soon — as a patient.

It didn't take me long to realize what risk factor I had overlooked. As a busy cardiologist who traveled a lot and worked long hours, stress was a constant part of my life. It was the factor I had failed to see.

These days, stress usually is included on the list of the major risk factors for heart disease. But most cardiologists give it short attention. I know better now.

But there are other risk factors that we often overlook — either because they don't affect as many people or because doctors are only now realizing how dangerous they are. These include:

1. Stress
2. Periodontal disease
3. Arthritis
4. Lupus
5. Sleep Apnea

6. Homocysteine (amino acid)
7. Low Hormone Levels

If you have any of these risk factors, you must pay attention to them and take the actions I set out to mitigate their impact on your heart. If you do not, the result could be deadly.

Risk 1: Stress Releases 'Fight-or-Flight' Hormones

Stress is the body's instinctive response to the perception of a threat. When we sense danger, our adrenal glands spring into action, and release a flood of hormones, including adrenalin and cortisol, into the bloodstream.

These hormones quicken the heartbeat and raise blood pressure, pumping additional blood to our arms and legs. That's why this is called the "fight-or-flight" response — because that added burst of blood gives us the temporary strength to either fight or flee.

Unfortunately, cortisol also fuels inflammation, the process that sets the stage for coronary artery disease.

Our bodies respond the same way to stress if it is temporary or chronic. For instance, whether we are faced with real sudden danger, such as having to swerve to avoid a car accident; or an ongoing stress, like staying awake all night worrying about unpaid bills, the effect on the body is largely the same.

So if you are under stress, you have to do something to alleviate it. If your job or occupation is the problem, think strongly about making a change. But if you can't get rid of the source of your stress, you can do other things to make your lifestyle as heart-healthy as possible.

• Eat healthy foods
• Schedule frequent work breaks
• Learn to relax

Personally, I have found that prayer and belonging to my religious community help me deal with the stresses I encounter; you might find that comforting as well.

Remember, stress kills people every day — and the kind of stress doesn't matter.

Risk 2: Gum Disease Spreads Bacteria Into the Arteries

Cardiologists hardly ever look inside their patients' mouths. But when I treated heart transplant patients at the Medical College of

Virginia's VA hospital in the late '80s and early '90s, I always checked their teeth and gums.

We don't yet know *exactly* how gum disease affects the heart, but we're beginning to get a pretty good idea.

First, all people have millions of bacteria living in their mouths. When a person has gum disease, that bacteria can get in the bloodstream through open sores. These bacteria then stick to plaque in coronary arteries, making the narrowing and inflammation even worse.

Another potential link focuses on the body's inflammatory response. When you have gum disease, your body is in a chronic, inflammatory state, which contributes to the likelihood atherosclerotic plaque will form.

In addition, when your arteries become inflamed, it's more likely that newly formed, soft plaque will rupture and create a blood clot that blocks an artery completely, leading to a heart attack.

So you must pay attention to your teeth in order to protect your heart! This means brushing your teeth after every meal, flossing daily, and regularly visiting the dentist.

Risk 3: Rheumatoid Arthritis Produces Chronic Inflammation

Rheumatoid arthritis (RA) is an autoimmune disease, meaning that it arises from the normal biological process your body uses to fight off viruses or bacteria. In people with an autoimmune disease, the body mistakes normal tissue for a threat and attacks the healthy tissue along with the foreign bodies. Autoimmune diseases affect women far more often than men.

RA causes a progressive inflammation of the joints, especially in the hands. But RA also raises the risk of heart disease by about 50 percent, most likely because it creates a chronic inflammatory state in the body, just as gum disease does.

If you have RA, make sure your doctors are monitoring you for heart disease. Tell them about any possible symptoms.

In addition, practice heart-healthy habits such as eating a plant-based diet and exercising daily. If the pain from your RA keeps you from doing common exercises, talk to your doctor about alternatives such as swimming, which is easier on the joints.

You also should know that steroids, which are often prescribed for RA, can raise your risk for heart disease. According to the Mayo Clinic, natural alternatives to steroids include plant oils (made from the seeds of evening primrose, borage, and black currant) and fish oil.

Consult your doctor before starting any alternative treatment for RA.

Risk 4: Lupus Attacks the Whole Body

Like rheumatoid arthritis, lupus is an autoimmune disease caused by an overactive immune response in the body, producing chronic inflammation. However, unlike RA, which affects only the joints, lupus attacks the whole body, including:

- Skin
- Stomach
- Bones
- Heart
- Lungs
- Kidneys
- Eyes

People with lupus are more likely to have the other major coronary heart disease risk factors, including high blood pressure, high cholesterol, and diabetes. This comes partly from the side effects of the strong steroids used to treat the lupus. Patients also tend to be inactive, because lupus causes fatigue as well as joint and muscle pain.

In fact, heart problems are the leading cause of death for people who suffer from lupus.

If you have lupus, make sure your doctor monitors you for signs of coronary heart disease and do everything you can to reduce your risk factors, such as eating a plant-based diet, doing regular exercise, and getting proper treatment for high blood pressure and high cholesterol.

Talk to your doctor about how to limit the use of steroids.

Risk 5: Sleep Apnea Increases Blood Pressure

Sleep disorders are a hot topic these days, as research continues to discover that they contribute to heart problems. Among the most serious of these disorders is sleep apnea, a condition affecting 10 million to 20 million Americans, most of them men 65 or older. (Sleep apnea also can occur in younger people, especially if they are overweight or they smoke.)

The most common form of sleep apnea occurs because the upper airways become obstructed during sleep, causing breathing to stop sometimes hundreds of times a night.

This sudden drop in oxygen alarms the body, causing the release of the same "fight-or-flight" hormones that raise blood pressure, ignite inflammation, and make blood clots more likely.

In addition to coronary artery disease, recent research has linked sleep apnea to the kind of memory and thinking problems that occur as we age.

Many people who have sleep apnea are completely unaware of it. However, major symptoms are loud snoring and excessive daytime drowsiness.

If you suspect you have sleep apnea, you should be evaluated at a sleep disorder clinic. Beware, though: Sleep disorders are big business, so many clinics are popping up. Make sure you choose a clinic with a well-trained and certified staff.

Sleep apnea is also linked to being overweight; weight loss often will correct it.

Moderate to severe sleep apnea also can be corrected with a device called a Continuous Positive Airway Pressure device, or CPAP, which delivers just enough air pressure through a mask on the nose to keep the upper airway passages open.

The CPAP must be worn consistently, though, because the sleep apnea will return if you stop using it. Alternative devices are available for those who find the CPAP uncomfortable.

Risk 6: Too Much Homocysteine Damages Arteries

Our bodies produce the amino acid homocysteine when we metabolize another amino acid, methionine, found in protein-rich foods. The B-vitamins folic acid (folate), B6, and B12 then convert homocysteine into still other amino acids that the body uses.

So some homocysteine in the blood is good. The normal level of homocysteine in the blood is 5 to 15 micromoles per liter.

Homocysteine made headlines a few years ago when studies indicated that too much of this amino acid in the blood could damage artery linings, increasing the risk of coronary artery disease and possibly accelerating the formation of blood clots.

However, subsequent studies did not see a link between homocysteine and increased heart disease — so the question remains.

Still, to be safe, you might want to have your homocysteine level checked. If it is too high (30 to100 micromoles per liter is considered moderately high; more than 100 micromoles per liter is severe), you should consider taking a supplement of folic acid along with vitamins B6 and B12 to lower your homocysteine.

Risk 7: Hormones Are Necessary for Heart Health

For Men: Testosterone levels peak in men in early adulthood and begin to decline after the age of 30. Research has long indicated that normal levels (250 to 850 ng/dl) are necessary to maintain good health, and that levels that are too high or too low are linked to coronary heart disease.

Not surprisingly, older men have lower testosterone levels than younger men — as many as 30 percent of men older than 75 have levels that are *much* lower than normal.

Men with very low levels of testosterone not only carry an increased risk of heart disease but also face loss of sexual function, decreased muscle mass, fatigue, and more.

In addition, men who develop anemia because their bone marrow is suppressed for various reasons, such as congestive heart failure, can benefit from testosterone replacement.

Testosterone supplements can be injected or administered transdermally with the use of a topical gel (once a day) or a patch that remains on the skin. Doses vary, so consult your doctor to determine the correct dosage for you.

However, beware of doctors hawking hormone replacement as an anti-aging "miracle cure."

For Women: Estrogen

Whether post-menopausal women should receive estrogen replacement therapy is an issue that has seesawed over the years. Years ago, the answer was simple: Yes.

Because the risk of heart disease in women rose as their estrogen declined, estrogen replacement seemed the obvious solution.

But then came some large-scale medical studies that cast doubt upon that conclusion. Use of estrogen replacement has dropped off since then. Now, the pendulum seems to be swinging back the other way.

Over the years, as I've watched my patients, the ones who seem to do the best are the ones who have well-balanced hormone levels. So, if your estrogen level is low, work with your doctor to weigh the benefits versus your individual risks.

Although this seems like a lengthy list of "Hidden Risk Factors," remember that the same common steps that help protect your heart, including eating right, quitting smoking, and becoming more active, can help resolve many of these factors.

If you have any conditions that heighten your risk of heart disease, taking action now can not only preserve your heart health, it could save your life.

CHAPTER 4

The Diabetes-Heart
Disease Connection

Here's a revelation that just might surprise you: Diabetes is a cardiovascular disease. No less an authority than the American Heart Association makes this somewhat surprising claim.

But diabetes is both a specific illness and a big part of the heart disease picture. In fact, diabetes contributes more to the development of cardiovascular disease and coronary heart ailments than any other risk factor besides smoking. The unhappy truth is that if you have diabetes and live long enough, you're almost sure to develop some form of heart disease.

In the United States, diabetes has grown to epidemic proportions, with the number of diagnosed cases having tripled since 1980. The American Diabetes Association now estimates that there are as many as 24 million Americans living with diabetes — that's 8 percent of the population. Of those cases, 18 million people have been officially diagnosed, while 6 million remain undiagnosed.

What's more, "pre-diabetes" — a condition in which the risk factors for diabetes are clearly present, though the disease itself has yet to develop — affects some 57 million people in the U.S.

The numbers also are skyrocketing among children: 151,000 people below the age of 20 currently have the disease, and statistics suggest that one in three children living today will have diabetes at some point.

How Diabetes Attacks Your Body

There are two types of diabetes: Type 1 and Type 2.

Type 1 diabetes — also called juvenile diabetes — is caused by the destruction of specific cells in the hormone-producing regions of the pancreas called the Langerhans islets. Despite extensive research, science is still not sure what causes these cells to be destroyed, though theories include everything from a virus to an as-yet unidentified autoimmune disease.

There are about 1 million of these Langerhans islets in a healthy adult pancreas. The Beta cells (or B cells) of the Langerhans secrete the hormone insulin directly into the bloodstream.

Insulin promotes tissue growth and keeps tissues from breaking down in the muscles, liver, and fat cells. Most importantly, insulin increases cells' ability to absorb glucose (sugar), thus providing energy. The amount of sugar in the blood drops as insulin performs its function.

Insulin also regulates fat storage in fat cells, as well as the total quantity of protein in the body. Without insulin, the body simply cannot function — at least not for long.

In Type 1 diabetes, the Langerhans islet B cells cease to produce insulin, and the body loses its ability to metabolize sugar — and its ability to feed the body's cells with glucose.

Eventually, that unabsorbed sugar begins to build up in the bloodstream like a thick syrup. The body reacts by causing the diabetic to feel thirsty in an effort to dilute the high sugar content of the blood. The person drinks constantly and, as a result, urinates frequently.

The diabetic also feels hungry all of the time, as the body cries out for the glucose that is not getting to the cells. Yet, despite eating more and more, rapid weight loss can occur as the cells starve and tissues literally shrink. Chronic fatigue sets in, along with irritability and blurred vision.

The body will then start burning fat for energy, and acids called ketones will build up in the bloodstream. This condition is known as ketoacidosis. At this point, the skin may become dry or flushed, and the diabetic can experience nausea, vomiting, or abdominal pain. He or she could have difficulty breathing and their breath may acquire a fruity odor.

If left untreated, the victim of Type 1 diabetes will become mentally confused and eventually go into a coma that can lead to death. Diabetes is serious business.

Type 2: The Hidden Diabetes
In Type 2 diabetes, the B cells of the pancreas continue to produce insulin, but at a slower rate. Also, the body's insulin receptors make use of insulin less efficiently over time.

This can set up a vicious cycle in which the body tries to compensate by producing more and more insulin, and the receptors become increasingly resistant to it. As a result, blood sugar levels climb and the unused insulin causes arterial walls and vascular tissues to thicken and become obstructed.

Most people who contract Type 2 diabetes do so later in life, typically in their 50s or 60s, and experience few if any immediate symptoms. Patients understand that Type 1 diabetes is serious, but they are often reluctant to accept that Type 2 — or late-onset — diabetes is a life-threatening disease.

As with Type 1, Type 2 diabetics may become thirsty and urinate more often, experience an increase in appetite, and gain or lose weight. The presence of these symptoms at the onset of Type 2 diabetes is uncommon, however. The Type 2 diabetic may also have become habituated to his symptoms over the course of a long time, drinking sodas throughout the day and taking his large appetite for normal.

Most often, patients don't realize there is a problem until they visit a doctor and receive negative test results. For instance, their blood work may come back with a fasting glucose value above 126, or their two-hour glucose tolerance test registers a value greater than 200, or their A1C test comes back above 6.5. All of these readings are signs of late-onset diabetes.

Still, for many patients this can seem a small concern   just a case of one too many pieces of pie. Ironically, denial of the condition is more frequent among those who actually have the best chance of avoiding full-blown Type 2 diabetes.

Many doctors tell their patients with fasting glucose values of 100 to 125, glucose tolerance values of 140 to 199, and A1C values greater than 6 that they are "pre-diabetic," meaning that they are especially at risk of developing Type 2 diabetes.

In my experience, almost no one in this category takes the diagnosis seriously enough.

Recent research indicates that patients with these "pre-diabetic" values will almost certainly develop Type 2 diabetes, and should be counseled and treated like patients who meet the official standards of diabetes in order to get them started on a course of treatment and lifestyle change. This is what I do in my practice.

So take note: If you are in this gray area, you are already in deep trouble and you deserve to know it! Your lifestyle has to change radically and immediately. Once you understand the way in which diabetes supercharges the heart disease engine, I think you'll agree.

Diabetes Kills the Cardiovascular 'Tree'

With Type 2 diabetes, we need to keep one thing clearly in mind: Insulin is a growth hormone. As long as the body is producing insulin, high blood sugar counts cause relatively little damage. It's the body's attempt to bring these counts down by producing more insulin that causes the damage.

Perhaps you've heard that diabetics can have trouble with their eyes, their kidneys, and the healing of wounds or ulcers, especially on their feet. The reason is that, in these areas, blood flows through extremely small vessels.

The kidneys, for example, are a vast network of tiny vessels called arterioles and capillaries, many of which are so small that only one blood cell can pass through them at a time.

What happens then when excess insulin causes the walls of these vessels to thicken? They quickly become blocked. Once a vessel is blocked, it dies. That's why the circulatory system of a person with uncontrolled diabetes looks like a dying tree. All the tiny buds at the ends of the branches disappear, then the shoots from which the buds would have sprouted, then the smallest branches, and so on.

When I look at someone with advanced diabetes, the patient's main arteries may look fine, but thousands upon thousands of the system's smallest branches have simply disappeared. The "tree" of a diabetic's circulatory system has become nothing but a trunk and a few denuded branches.

What's more, that vast network of small vessels in the kidneys is actually used to filter waste products out of the blood. When this no longer functions, the diabetic needs to go on dialysis treatment — that is, they need to have their blood filtered by a machine.

Eye and foot problems are caused by the same withering of the cardiovascular system. When the body can't supply enough blood flow to the rods and cones of the eye, these tissues die and the person can become blind.

Likewise, when a diabetic gets a sore on his foot, it can turn into an ulcer that refuses to heal because there's not enough blood supply to rebuild the tissue.

These conditions are rightly associated with diabetes, but their immediate cause is the destruction of the cardiovascular system. Diabetes and cardiovascular disease work together to deliver a 1-2 punch to the body's most vulnerable systems.

Metabolic Syndrome

Metabolic syndrome is the name for a condition that encompasses several risk factors for both cardiovascular disease and diabetes. These risk factors include:

- Insulin resistance
- Hypertension (high blood pressure)
- Hyperglycemia (elevated sugar blood counts)
- Dyslipidemia, or excess fats in the blood

At present, we do not fully understand the link between hypertension and diabetes, though evidence is growing that they do not simply occur together but are causally related. We do know, however, that high blood pressure makes nephropathy (damage to, or disease in the kidneys) much worse.

The elevated dyslipidemia (high levels of blood fats) that we are most concerned about has three distinct characteristics:

1. Elevated very-low-density lipoproteins (VLDL)

2. Small low-density lipoprotein (LDL) particles that are now being described in testing as Pattern B LDL particles

3. Low levels of high-density-lipoprotein (HDL) cholesterol. This triad is described as an "atherogenic" condition, meaning that together these characteristics generate atherosclerosis, or hardening of the arteries through plaque deposits.

Often, diabetics do not have very high LDL counts. Still, these counts are high enough to generate atherosclerosis. Aggressively pushing LDL cholesterol levels down reduces the risk of coronary artery disease events in patients with diabetes.

Researchers have also found that people with metabolic syndrome experience changes in the way their blood coagulates, and are prone to forming clots in response to plaque deposits in the arteries. The rupture of these blood clots is the most common way heart attacks and strokes occur.

With the same risk factors generating both cardiovascular disease and Type 2 diabetes — and both of these factors leading to hardening of the arteries and the formation of plaque deposits and blood clots — diabetes and cardiovascular disease wreak exactly the type of damage that leads to heart attacks and strokes.

So if you have elevated blood sugar counts, elevated VLDL counts, Pattern B LDL, low levels of HDL, and hypertension, you'd better beware: Full-blown Type 2 diabetes is right around the corner.

Indeed, any two of these predisposing risk factors are cause for serious concern.

What You Can Do

It's true that there are other factors contributing to diabetes about which a person can do little. Age, genetic inheritance, sex, and, to a degree, race all play a factor. (Hispanics and Native Americans are more inclined to diabetes than the rest of the population).

Type 2 diabetes can often be cured by changing lifestyle: a good diet, consistent exercise, and weight loss will all minimize the symptoms. The first key to ducking the 1-2 punch of Type 2 diabetes and heart disease is to change the way you eat.

A diet that concentrates on fresh fruit and vegetables, lean meats, and whole grain breads will go a long way toward lowering your risk.

The best exercise is walking one hour per day. You can also play tennis, go ballroom dancing, ride a bicycle, or work in the garden. Your goal should be to elevate your heart rate for an extended period of time. A good rule of thumb is that, when exercising, you should always be able to talk. That's a sign that the exercise is "aerobic," meaning that your system has all the oxygen it needs.

Over the course of six months, lifestyle change that results in substantial weight loss will also have a dramatic effect on your lipid profile — that is, the fats in your blood.

Another key is to work with — not against — your doctor. Develop a plan along with him or her to put diabetes behind you as soon as possible, and for the rest of your life.

Don't be afraid to take the medications your doctor prescribes as a bridge to hitting target values for cholesterol and blood sugar. And let your doctor know, in no uncertain terms, that you intend to beat this disease and get off medication as soon as possible.

Keep every appointment. Insist on seeing your blood work and knowing what each count means. Start with a target date on which you will achieve your ideal body weight, and keep track of your progress in a journal. Weigh yourself daily and record your progress.

I like to start my patients on diet and exercise programs right away, and see how much they can accomplish in one month's time. Our practice has set up a "metabolic clinic" to provide as much help with these lifestyle changes as possible.

If the testing values of my patients don't come back into line quickly enough, however, I will prescribe medications. Diabetes and cardiovascular disease are such a devastating combination that I treat diabetics and even "pre-diabetics" as aggressively as possible.

Finally, stress reduction is a key factor. If you have Type 2 diabetes or are pre-diabetic, you have to understand that a battle has already begun. You must change your lifestyle now — and exercise will help with controlling stress.

The discipline of exercise should be combined with the discipline of a regular daily schedule. It's important that you eat three meals a day; never skip breakfast. Plan your snacks — such as a handful of almonds or walnuts — to bridge the hungry hours between meals.

Go out to eat as little as possible because controlling what you eat away from home is extremely difficult. American restaurants offer customers more food on a single plat than two people should eat.

Finally, enlist your loved ones in the battle. It may be hard for them to understand how much diabetes is threatening your life. After all, to them you look fine, even if you are a little overweight. They can help you start your life anew, free of diabetes and the heart disease that will eventually come with it.

CHAPTER 5

Stroke Warnings Can Save Your Life

What is a stroke and how do you recognize it when you are having one? If you can't answer that question, you're not alone. A recent telephone survey of 71,000 adults in 13 states asked respondents to identify the five warning signs of a stroke and what people should do if they thought they might be having one. Only one in six people got the right answers.

I have discovered the same thing in my own practice: Most of my patients don't know what the symptoms of a stroke are, or what actions to take when they experience them.

My definition of a stroke is this: It's a heart attack in the brain. And it can have devastating consequences. Not only is stroke the third leading cause of death in the United States, it is the No. 1 cause of serious, long-term disability.

Stroke is a life-threatening emergency. Time is critical. This is truly a case where every minute counts. That's why it's so important to know the warning signs.

A stroke occurs when there is a sudden interruption of blood supply to the brain. There are two types of major stroke: ischemic strokes and hemorrhagic strokes.

The most common type of stroke, an ischemic stroke, occurs in 87 percent of all cases. This is the type of stroke that is much like a heart attack in the brain. The term "ischemic" means lack of blood supply, usually due to a clot in a vessel that supplies blood. When this happens, oxygen and other nutrients cannot get to the brain. The clot can be one of two types:

- An embolus is a blood clot that forms in another part of the body, then breaks off and travels toward the brain, where it becomes lodged in the smaller vessels, forming a blockage.

• A thrombus is a stationary clot that forms in an artery that supplies blood to the brain. This type of blockage does not move, but as it grows it blocks more and more blood flow to the tissues of the brain.

Ischemic strokes are treated with blood thinners and clot-busting medications.

A hemorrhagic stroke occurs when a blood vessel ruptures in the brain. This can happen as the result of persistent high blood pressure or an aneurysm — a weakness in the wall of a blood vessel.

When the vessel breaks, blood seeps into sensitive brain tissue surrounding the rupture. Damage can occur either from the presence of the blood itself or because of the buildup of pressure within the cranium, which presses brain tissue against the inside of the skull.

Hemorrhagic strokes can cause damage very quickly, and may require surgery to stop the bleeding as well as follow-up with medication.

Risk Factors for Stroke

Your first line of defense in preventing a stroke is to know where you stand. So before we get into the actual warning signs for a stroke, let's review some of the risk factors. Controlling these factors is not a guarantee against a stroke, of course, but it can lower the chances considerably.

Statistics show that up to 50 percent of all strokes are preventable.

Everyone has two kinds of risk factors — those they can change and those they cannot. Here's a rundown:

The things you can't change

• **Age.** The risk of stroke increases with age. Two-thirds of strokes happen in people over the age of 65. The chance of having a stroke almost doubles for each decade of life after age 55.

• **Race.** Those with higher risk of stroke include African Americans, Native Americans, and Alaskan Natives. African Americans have twice the risk of a first ischemic stroke because they have a higher incidence of hypertension and diabetes.

• **Gender.** Stroke is about 25 percent more common in men than women until age 75. Overall, however, more women than men die of stroke. Birth control pills and pregnancy pose particular risks for younger women. And because women live longer than men, they are more likely to have an increased death rate after age 75.

- **Family History.** Your risk is higher if a parent, grandparent, or sibling has had a stroke. This includes the mini-stroke called a transient ischemic attack (TIA).

- **Personal History.** Anyone who has had a prior stroke, TIA, or a heart attack has a much higher risk of another stroke. A TIA is a very strong predictor of a stroke. Those who have had a TIA have about 10 times greater risk for a subsequent stroke — which is why TIAs are also called "warning strokes."

The things you can change

- **Hypertension.** High blood pressure is by far the most significant risk factor for stroke. Luckily, this biggest risk factor is one that you can control. It can be managed with lifestyle changes and medication.

- **High Cholesterol.** High levels of bad (LDL) cholesterol can result in hardening of the arteries, which leads to plaque deposits on the walls of blood vessels.

- **Stress.** Studies show that people who experience high stress levels are more likely to develop hardened arteries than those who stay calm under pressure. The reason for this is that high stress causes the body to release more cortisol (the "fight or flight" hormone), which causes arteries to narrow.

- **Food and Alcohol Choices.** Diets high in saturated fats and trans fats raise cholesterol levels, while diets high in salt increase blood pressure. These two factors together can put a great deal of strain on blood vessels and the heart. A moderate amount of alcohol has a protective effect, but alcohol abuse increases risk of stroke.

- **Smoking.** The combination of nicotine and carbon monoxide in cigarette smoke (including secondhand smoke) is extremely damaging to the cardiovascular system. Over time, it causes a narrowing and weakening of the arteries (atherosclerosis). This results in a need for the heart to pump harder, leading to hypertension. Smoking combined with the use of oral contraceptives greatly increases the risk of stroke in women.

- **Sedentary Lifestyle and Obesity.** Being inactive increases your weight, which leads to an increase in blood pressure.

- **Diabetes.** With diabetes comes serious circulation problems that can double the risk of stroke. Also, many people with diabetes have other risk factors, such as being overweight and having high blood pressure and/or high cholesterol.

- **Heart Disease.** The same problems that are associated with heart disease (narrowing of the arteries, plaque buildup, etc.) can lead to stroke. That's why I call stroke a heart attack in the brain.

The Five Major Stroke Warning Signs

If your first line of defense in preventing a stroke is assessing your personal health, your second — and even more important — defense is recognizing the warning signs. This is what will save your life if you're headed for a stroke.

There are five main warning signs of a stroke. You might experience some or all of them.

1. Sudden vision problems; difficulty seeing out of one or both eyes.

2. Sudden headache; severe pain with no apparent cause.

3. Sudden confusion; you become unable to think or speak clearly, or can't understand what others are saying to you.

4. Sudden numbness; weakness and lack of feeling in the face, arm, or leg, particularly if it is isolated on one side of the body.

5. Sudden lack of coordination, including dizziness or loss of balance.

The warning signs of a stroke are very much like the warning signs along a road. They're there to alert you to a danger you might not see coming. But if you take heed, you can avoid calamity.

An even more serious warning sign of an impending stroke is something called a transient ischemic attack (TIA) or "mini-stroke." About one-third of the people who experience a TIA go on to have a major stroke within a year, according to the American Stroke Association. This is the most important warning sign to recognize because taking it seriously gives you time to prevent a more serious stroke.

Basically, there is no difference between a TIA and a stroke except for duration and damage. In layman's terms, a transient ischemic attack simply means a temporary interruption of blood flow (and oxygen) to the brain.

It happens very quickly and lasts just a short time — between 1 to 5 minutes. And when it's over, there is no permanent damage to the brain. It is possible for the symptoms to last a couple of hours, but there is always complete recovery within 24 hours.

Because it happens so fast, many people are inclined to ignore it. In fact, the whole event barely takes enough time to wonder what on Earth just happened!

But a TIA is almost always the result of a clot, and therefore it's a serious warning signal.

Think of the aorta, the largest artery in the body, as a river from the heart to the brain. A blood clot that breaks loose is carried by that river into smaller and smaller pathways until it reaches a place too narrow to pass. At that point, it becomes a blockage cutting off blood flow to the brain.

If the clot dislodges right away or the body dissolves it, the symptoms will be temporary — a TIA. But whatever caused the event is still lurking within the cardiovascular system. The incident may have passed, but the danger has not.

Not surprisingly, half of the people who experience a TIA fail to report it to their doctor. But they're walking time bombs, even if they don't know it.

TIAs also can occur after a patient has experienced a full-blown stroke. If this happens, it means something in the treatment plan is not working. In this case, the patient should seek medical attention immediately.

I call a TIA "the first shot in battle" when it comes to stroke prevention treatment. It's not a warning you can afford to ignore. Taking it seriously and getting immediate help can save your life.

Time is your best ally against a stroke. The biggest mistakes people make when they experience a TIA or other stroke warning signs are denial, indecision, and waiting too long to get help.

If you can get to the hospital right away, doctors can get the arteries opened up with medication or surgery. Often, the stroke can be stopped in its tracks so that damage is reduced or even reversed.

In addition to recognizing the warning signs, it is important to call 911 and get a paramedic on the scene as soon as possible. Do not try to drive yourself or a loved one to the hospital. You will only waste precious time.

Paramedics have a specific protocol in place for stroke patients. They are obligated to take you to a designated stroke hospital, and will call ahead with a "stroke alert." This means the hospital will begin to assemble a qualified team in the emergency room while you are still on the way. That's the level of urgency required for stroke care.

Once in the hospital, a stroke patient immediately will be given a neurological exam and be sent for a CT scan of the brain. That will determine if the cause is bleeding or a clot. If it's a clot — as it usually is — additional tests will be performed to determine the location of the clot, then a blood thinner can be administered.

All of this needs to happen quickly to limit damage.

Finland: A Case Study in Stroke Prevention

You should never believe that stroke or heart attack is inevitable. In fact, that's what they used to think in Finland, a country that in the 1960s had the world's highest death rate from heart disease and stroke.

Then, in 1972, the government launched a prevention program. Everyone from doctors and nurses to officials in libraries and schools was asked to promote a healthy lifestyle. Schools improved lunch programs and local governments built walking tracks, pools, and ice rinks.

The message from the government was to quit smoking, reduce dietary fat and salt, get adequate exercise, and eat plenty of fresh fruits and vegetables. People were also encouraged to monitor their blood pressure and cholesterol.

Finnish families took the message seriously, mostly because they had been directly affected by heart attacks and strokes. And the media got in on the program, too. One Finnish doctor produced a television show that encouraged 10 contestants to lower their blood pressure and cholesterol. The show was so popular that it ran for 15 years and inspired many of the country's cities to sponsor similar competitions of their own.

The end result? Since the early 1970s, the incidence of heart attack and stroke has fallen 75 to 80 percent in Finland.

I was able to observe this amazing turnaround firsthand on a visit to Finland last year. I traveled throughout the entire country while speaking on a ministry tour, and I was repeatedly impressed by the fitness level of the Finnish people.

An estimated 65 percent of Finns are regularly active because they have so many sports/exercise facilities available. Every city and village has well-lit, well-maintained paths for walking, biking, and cross-country skiing. Fruit and vegetable consumption has tripled since the 1960s.

The Finns are remarkable proof that lifestyle changes can dramatically affect your quality of life. In fact, *Newsweek* recently ranked Finland as the most desirable country in the world to live in.

Modern medicine has made tremendous strides in protecting and maintaining our health — and preventing and treating stroke is just one example. I'm most aware of that when I travel to a Third World country where medical care is severely limited. I am committed to providing medicine and healing in whatever way I can, but it is certainly a lot easier in this part of the world.

Time is critical for the salvage and recovery of brain function. The longer you wait, the more brain tissue you will lose. And the sooner you get treatment, the sooner damage can be reversed.

I cannot stress enough the importance of identifying the warning signs of a stroke. If any of those signs occur in you or a companion, don't delay in getting help. If you're in doubt, call 911.

With knowledge and good medical care on your side, you can prevent or survive a stroke and go on with the rest of your life.

CHAPTER 6

What You Need to Know

Congestive heart failure is perhaps the most challenging of all the conditions a cardiologist has to treat. Why? Because successful treatment requires time and patience, two things doctors often lack. As a result, patients often are treated and monitored inadequately.

Many times, people diagnosed with congestive heart failure — also often called simply "heart failure" — begin a rapid downward slide. They feel bad all the time and spend years going in and out of the hospital. Eventually, their lives are cut short.

According to the Centers for Disease Control and Prevention, heart failure is a contributing cause in nearly 300,000 deaths in the United States every year. But this does not have to happen! For years, we've known how to treat heart failure successfully. The problem is that we don't.

In June of 2011, the *American Heart Journal* published a study reporting that if cardiologists followed national heart treatment guidelines, 68,000 people could be saved each year. The American Heart Association issued a similar warning two years ago.

Actually, heart failure is not really a disease, but the name given to what occurs when your heart becomes too weak to pump the amount of blood your body needs.

Treating heart failure is like solving a puzzle. It's fascinated me since early in my career, when I treated many heart failure patients as director of the Medical College of Virginia's VA heart transplant program. That's why I'm so eager to share the latest information on this condition.

To comprehend what happens with heart failure, you must understand how the heart works. It is a four-chambered muscle with a two-sided pumping system — one on the right and the other on the left. The right side pumps blood into the lungs to fill with oxygen, and then the left side takes over, delivering the blood to the rest of your body.

Your heart also depends on a series of four valves — the aortic, pulmonary, tricuspid, and mitral valves — that open and close along with the muscle contractions, keeping the blood flowing forward in the right direction.

In addition, the heart has its own electrical system, which synchronizes its pumping action so the blood moves in a steady fashion.

The Vicious Cycle

When the heart is forced to work too hard for a long time, it can become too weak to pump blood throughout the body. The body tries to compensate by producing a series of structural changes, a process called "remodeling." This helps in the short run — but over time, it is harmful.

With remodeling, the heart is forced to hold more blood; it becomes enlarged. As a result, some of the blood backs up into the lungs, which causes congestion that comes with heart failure.

When this happens, the body reduces the blood supply flowing to the kidneys, which regulate fluids. This causes excess fluid buildup, resulting in the swelling that is often seen in the legs and ankles of patients with heart failure.

The more fluid buildup there is, the harder the heart has to work — and that weakens it even further. It's a vicious cycle.

Heart failure usually occurs in people older than 65. However, even if you're younger than that, if you have one or more of these conditions, you're at risk:

- **Coronary Artery Disease.** This occurs when your heart's coronary arteries become narrowed. The good news is that procedures are available that can restore blood flow. These include balloon angioplasty or stenting (the use of a balloon/stent to widen the coronary artery) and coronary bypass surgery (the grafting of a vessel to create an alternative blood flow around a blockage).

- **Heart attack.** When one of the coronary arteries is not just narrowed but becomes blocked, this interruption in blood flow to the heart results in a heart attack. If the heart muscle is damaged, it tries to repair itself. In doing so, it becomes weaker, often setting the stage for heart failure.

- **High Blood Pressure.** Blood pressure measures how hard the heart is working to pump blood throughout the body. High blood pressure shows that the heart is working too hard, which puts it under the kind of strain that can lead to heart failure.

- **Diabetes.** This metabolic disorder, which leads to the buildup of too much sugar in your blood, also may lead to a condition called "diabetic cardiomyopathy," which is an enlarged and weakened heart caused by the rapid progression of coronary disease.

- **Valvular Disease.** As we age, the valves of the heart can become stiff or "stenotic." The valves then cannot close or open properly and can become leaky, making blood flow difficult and requiring the heart to work harder. Valve replacement or repair may be necessary.

- **Arrhythmias.** Problems with the heart's electrical system can give rise to irregular heartbeats, called arrhythmias. "Atrial fibrillation" and "sick sinus syndrome" are the two types of arrhythmias that can trigger heart failure. With atrial fibrillation, the upper chamber of the heart begins quivering uncontrollably, instead of contracting normally. Sick sinus syndrome is a condition that causes the heart to beat slowly.

Symptoms of Heart Failure

The symptoms of heart failure can come on suddenly, which is called "acute heart failure." However, the symptoms more often appear gradually, a condition that is labeled "chronic heart failure."

People with chronic heart failure often end up in the hospital before they even realize something is seriously wrong. Take my patient Ron, for example. He noticed he was becoming short of breath and coughing, so he called his doctor.

"Don't worry, it sounds like you've got the upper respiratory infection that's going around. I'll give you an antibiotic," his doctor told him.

Ron took the drug, but his condition got worse. By the weekend, he was in my emergency room, struggling to breathe. If Ron's doctor had listened to his lungs and heard a sound called "rales" (which sound like a clicking, rattling, or bubbling in the lungs), it would have indicated that Ron's congestion was caused by heart failure and not an upper respiratory infection.

Other symptoms of heart failure include:

- Shortness of breath and difficulty breathing with mild exertion or while sleeping. Having to sleep propped up in bed or in a chair is a telltale sign.

- Profound fatigue that makes even walking a block exhausting.

- Persistent coughing or wheezing.

- Rapid weight gain and/or body swelling, which usually occurs in the legs and ankles.

- Rapid heartbeat or palpitations.

- Lack of appetite, nausea.

- Angina (chest pain) if you've had a heart attack or are newly diagnosed with heart disease.

If you have heart failure and you notice new symptoms, worsening of symptoms, or your symptoms return, call your doctor.

Heart failure progresses rapidly, so prompt treatment can save a trip to the hospital.

Drug Treatment Options

Heart failure treatment often requires several drugs, and it is of utmost importance that you take each exactly as directed. Make sure you have detailed, written instructions for each drug, along with what to watch for so you can alert your doctor to any adverse side effects.

Here are a few of the drugs your doctor might suggest:

- **Diuretics.** Years ago, diuretics were the only treatment we had to treat heart failure. They eliminated the body's excess fluid but did nothing to improve the heart function. Diuretics are still a mainstay of heart failure treatment, but they now are used in combination with other medications that strengthen the heart.

- **Angiotensin-Converting Enzyme Inhibitors (ACE inhibitors).** These drugs were the "game-changer" that transformed heart failure from a condition that had to be lived with to one that was actually reversible. ACE inhibitors not only relieve symptoms, but also actually strengthen the heart by blocking the effects of angiotensin II, a hormone the kidneys produce. Inhibiting this hormone causes blood vessels to relax, which lowers blood pressure, so the heart doesn't have to work so hard.

- **Beta-Blockers.** This class of drugs usually is given in conjunction with ACE inhibitors. They work by lowering blood pressure and pulse rate, which improves the heart's ability to relax. This, over time, improves the heart's pumping ability. Beta-blockers also assist in a favorable remodeling of the heart back to its normal state.

- **Digoxin.** This drug strengthens the force of the heart's contractions, which helps restore a steady heartbeat and reverses heart failure.

- **Vasodilators/Nitrates.** These are another type of drug that treats heart failure by relaxing the blood vessels so the blood can flow forward more easily. Usually, they are prescribed for people who can't take ACE inhibitors.

Successful heart failure treatment restores the body's harmony. Think of your body as an orchestra. When a key member of the orchestra (the heart) begins to falter, the rest of the orchestra has to work harder to compensate. This throws everything out of sync, and before long all you have is a jumble of noise instead of music. The conductor (your doctor) steps in to restore order. Then, with all the musicians in sync again, harmony is restored. Fortunately, nowadays, we have more ways than ever to restore harmony.

If you have heart failure, expect to be taking at least two different types of drugs, and usually more.

Surgical Treatment Options

If an arrhythmia is causing heart failure, a doctor might recommend a pacemaker or implantable cardioverter defibrillator (ICD) to regulate your heartbeat.

"Dual-chambered pacemakers" are usually used to treat heart failure. These have two leads, or wires, one each attached to the upper and lower chambers of the heart, which synchronize the heartbeat and improve blood flow and heart function.

A defibrillator monitors the heart's rhythm; when it senses an arrhythmia, it delivers a shock that reverts the heart to its normal rhythm. These are reserved for people with serious heart failure whose ejection fraction — a measure of the output of blood pumped from the right and left ventricles — has fallen below 35 percent, putting them at risk of a life-threatening arrhythmia.

Before the development of today's treatments, a heart transplant was the only hope for people with the most severe cases of heart failure. A heart transplant is still an option, but is rarely performed because of all the other effective tools we have now.

People with heart failure serious enough to require a transplant may be given a device called an LVAD (left ventricular assist device). An LVAD is a set of two small battery-operated pumps, which are implanted in the body and powered by an external controller worn on the belt. You may have heard of an LVAD because former Vice President Dick Cheney was given one in 2010.

The successful treatment of heart failure also depends on reregulating the way your body handles fluids. Your doctor plays an important role, but much of the responsibility in making sure your body does not become waterlogged rests on your following these important recommendations every day:

- **Restrict Your Salt Intake.** Salt causes your body to retain fluid, so you need to limit intake to less than one teaspoon per day.

- **Watch Your Fluid Intake.** More fluid in your blood vessels means your heart has to pump harder. You can tell whether your body is collecting fluid by weighing yourself daily. If you're experiencing swelling, cut back on your fluid consumption.

- **Keep Track of Your Weight.** Excess water weight can be a tipoff to a worsening in your condition. Weigh yourself each morning before you eat or drink anything, and call your doctor if you've gained 3 pounds or more.

If you have heart failure, your care should be in the hands of a trained cardiologist. Many medical institutions have centers devoted to heart failure treatment, so you can find a good doctor there.

The most important message is that heart failure can be reversed. It takes work and commitment, but it can be done.

CHAPTER 7

Don't Let Your Heart Valves Ruin Your Golden Years

Everyone is familiar with the sound that a heartbeat makes. It happens in two parts: an initial, softer thump followed by a louder beat — "lub-DUB, lub-DUB."

This sequence occurs approximately 100,000 times a day for your whole life. Though you might think that the sound comes from the heart muscle contracting, it's actually the valves closing inside the chambers of the heart that creates that familiar sound.

But problems can arise with these heart valves due to everyday wear. After all, 100,000 beats each day is a lot of work. And with the population of the United States living longer and the baby boomers moving into their golden years, valvular heart disease is a mounting public health concern that we can't afford to ignore.

I like to tell my patients that the valves of the heart are like saloon doors. They swing open in a forward motion to let blood exit the heart, and then they slam shut to keep blood from flowing back into the heart chambers.

Each of the four chambers has a valve, and the valves work in pairs. That's why you get a two-part sound when blood is pumped from the heart.

The upper chambers of the heart are called the left and right atria; the lower chambers are the left and right ventricles.

Here's how the valves work:

1. The **tricuspid valve** lets blood out of the right atrium down into the right ventricle.

2. The **pulmonary valve** lets blood out of the right ventricle into pulmonary arteries so it can go to the lungs and pick up

oxygen. Pulmonary veins then bring oxygen-rich blood back to the left atrium.

3. The **mitral valve** lets blood out of the left atrium down into the left ventricle.

4. The **aortic valve** lets blood out of the left ventricle into the aorta — the largest artery in the body, which carries the blood to other arteries for delivery throughout the cardiovascular system.

These are the "saloon doors" that swing open and close as blood flows through. When the valves of the upper chambers release blood into the ventricles, you get the soft "lub" sound. When the valves of the lower chambers push blood from the heart out into the body, you get the harder "DUB" sound.

In a healthy functioning heart, each valve should open and close completely. When they don't, the blood doesn't flow as it should.

In addition, when things go wrong with the heart valves, they make different sounds that can be heard with a stethoscope. For instance, instead of the clean "lub-DUB," a doctor might hear a whooshing or a hissing along with the usual sounds. Or there could be other unusual rhythms and sounds. Some of these variations are harmless, but many are not.

Two main things can go wrong with the heart valves. If they don't open all the way, the path for blood flow becomes narrower. This narrowing is called "stenosis." Imagine if one of the saloon doors doesn't open, or only opens part way — then you would have to squeeze through sideways.

The other problem occurs when a valve doesn't close all the way. When this happens, blood leaks back into the chamber, making more work for the heart. This leaking back into the chambers is called "regurgitation."

Blood flow that is unobstructed doesn't make any sound. However, when blood flow is impeded by narrowing or leaking it makes a distinctive sound known as a "murmur."

Quite often, murmurs can occur when there is nothing wrong with the heart. These are called "innocent" murmurs. On the other hand, when a murmur is abnormal it is a clear sign of valvular heart disease.

If your doctor thinks you have an abnormal heart murmur, additional tests will be ordered. A chest X-ray can reveal if your heart is enlarged, which is a sign that your heart may be working too hard because of stenosis or regurgitation.

An electrocardiogram (EKG) will record your heart rhythm to show the pattern of the heartbeat.

An echocardiogram can provide a clear picture of the heart valves to see what kind of shape they are in.

An innocent heart murmur doesn't need further treatment. But an abnormal one must be monitored. Certain medications offer specific benefits:

- Digitalis can help your heart squeeze harder if it is weak.

- Diuretics or ACE inhibitors can help with high blood pressure, which can worsen a heart murmur.

- Statins can help lower cholesterol, which seems to impact heart valves.

Symptoms of Valvular Heart Disease

There are many symptoms to look for if you think you may have valvular heart disease. You may find yourself to be short of breath, either when active or even while lying down. It may be necessary to sleep with your body propped up on pillows to enable easier breathing.

You may experience fatigue and dizziness or discomfort in your chest. Going out into cold air may feel uncomfortable. Palpitations and irregular heartbeat might be symptoms as well.

Swelling of lower legs, feet, and abdomen can occur and cause you to gain several pounds very quickly.

All of these things can be symptoms of the heart valves not working correctly. Valvular disease usually can be detected by listening to the heart sounds with a stethoscope. Do not put off having an examination if you have any of these symptoms.

Valvular disease is the leading cause of congestive heart failure, and it progresses with age.

Although there is little you can do on your own to reverse valvular disease, cholesterol management has been shown to slow the progression of aortic stenosis (narrowing of the aortic valve). To manage your cholesterol, eat fresh foods. In addition, here's a list of what *not* to eat to help keep cholesterol in check:

- Fatty cuts of meat, bacon, sausage, and processed meats

- High-fat dairy products, including butter, and egg yolks

- Processed grains like cookies, cakes, and pastries

- Coconut oil, palm oil, cocoa butter, lard, and shortening

I'm a firm believer that 85 percent of heart disease could be eliminated with the right lifestyle habits. That includes moderate alcohol consumption (or none at all), and no smoking.

Another important preventive measure is to get some exercise every day. At the very least, take a 30-minute walk several times a week.

As always, controlling the stress in your life is vital to heart health. One of the most effective ways to do this is to have a grateful attitude and a rich spiritual life.

Preventive measures are the best way to take care of your heart and protect its valves. In the course of 70 years, the average human heart beats more than 2.5 billion times, and with every beat, the "saloon door" valves have to control the flow of blood.

You can keep those doors in good working order with proper diet, exercise, and good stress management.

Living With Valvular Heart Disease

If you do find out that you have valvular heart disease, there are a number of things you can do to protect yourself from experiencing complications.

In the case of stenosis, blood pressure and cholesterol levels have to be kept under control. Less pressure in the arteries is easier on the valves.

For regurgitation, the medications prescribed — usually ACE inhibitors — are referred to as "after-load-reducing-agents" because they help a leaky valve work better. These medications reduce the backward pressure of the blood, allowing more forward blood flow.

Other measures that can help you avoid complications include:

- Take antibiotics before any surgical procedure.

- Take good care of your teeth and gums with regular dental visits.

- Take preventive antibiotics before any dental work or medical tests that involve bleeding, including major and minor surgery. You are at risk of an infection called endocarditis even if you've had a valve repair or replacement.

- Take medications such as diuretics, anti-arrhythmic medications, vasodilators, beta blockers, or anti-coagulants.

- Keep a list of your medications and let any doctor or dentist you visit know what you are taking and that you have valve disease.

General heart-healthy habits also apply even more significantly if you have valvular heart disease. Once again, a nutritious, plant-based diet is always the first thing I recommend.

Another thing you might do is carry an identification card that indicates that you have heart valve disease. This will help doctors to understand how best to treat you in case of a cardiac event.

You can get these cards from a doctor or download one from the American Heart Association. For more information, call the American Heart Association.

Surgical Treatments for Bad Heart Valves

The valves of the heart have to open and close 70 to 80 times a minute, every minute of every day. That results in a lot of wear and tear, and as people live longer, valvular heart disease will become more of an issue.

Once valve problems develop, you essentially have a mechanical problem with your heart. Medications can help relieve the pressure on the heart valves, but eventually a malfunctioning heart valve may need to be repaired or replaced. In some cases, a balloon procedure can be performed on a defective valve; this is very similar to opening a narrowed blood vessel.

If you learn that you or a loved one needs a heart valve repaired or replaced, the most important thing I can tell you is this: *Go to a hospital that specializes in treating valvular disease.*

A valve replacement must be done by a surgeon who has a long history of working on valves. This usually will be a more mature physician rather than a recent graduate or a surgeon who does only a few procedures per year.

Do not take this advice lightly. Go to a heart center or a university hospital that does a high volume of valve replacements.

There are two options for replacing a damaged heart valve. The first is a "tissue" valve, which comes from either a cow, a pig, or a human cadaver. This kind of valve does not require the patient to take anticoagulation (blood-thinner) treatment. These valves last about 10 years.

The other choice is a mechanical heart valve made of metal or plastic. This type of valve requires lifetime treatment with blood thinner medications in order to keep clots from forming on the valve. Taking blood thinners can be a problem for younger, more active people, but the valve will last forever.

One patient of mine, Frank, came to me about five years ago experiencing fatigue and shortness of breath. Testing showed that he had moderate aortic stenosis with a valve opening area of 1.1 square centimeters. A normal aortic valve opening is 3 to 4 square centimeters. Stenosis becomes critical when it goes below 1 square centimeter.

Frank had yearly echocardiograms to track progression of the valve disease. After five years, his aortic valve opening had narrowed to 0.4 square centimeters, and he had developed an irregular heartbeat due to the strain of the blocked valve.

A bovine tissue valve was used to replace Frank's narrowed aortic valve and he was able to leave the hospital in five days. Total recovery after a valve replacement is generally three months, and Frank was able to get back to his normal life, including flying his helicopter, within that time.

If you get a valve replacement of either kind, it is important to always be on the alert for endocarditis — an infection of the valves and parts of the inside lining of the heart muscle that occurs when bacteria are introduced into the bloodstream. This can happen during a dental procedure or any kind of surgery if you have a replacement heart valve. It is vital to take antibiotics prior to any such procedure to prevent this very serious infection of the heart.

You may not always be able to control what happens to your body as you age, but healthy lifestyle makes a big difference. Fortunately, if mechanical problems such as valvular heart disease do arise, modern medicine can treat them effectively.

CHAPTER 8

Chest Pain Warning Signals

Chest pain is one of the most frightening episodes a person can experience. No matter how it strikes — whether it wakes you at night, strikes suddenly during your daily routine, or sneaks up on you gradually over the course of several hours — you're likely to have only one thought: "Am I having a heart attack?"

Such a reaction is human nature. After all, coronary artery disease is the biggest killer of men and women around the world, and chest pain is its No. 1 warning sign.

However, chest pain is actually quite common and can have many causes other than heart attack. So how do you know if the pain you are feeling warrants a trip to the emergency room, or if it comes from another, possibly even a harmless, cause?

People who have coronary artery disease experience a type of chest pain known as angina pectoris, which is more commonly known simply as "angina." This type of pain occurs when the heart has to work extra hard to pump oxygen-rich blood to the rest of the body.

There are two types of angina, referred to as "stable" angina and "unstable" angina.

Stable angina occurs in people who have long-term heart disease; their coronary arteries are lined with plaque that has often calcified and is rock hard. This type of plaque is unlikely to rupture and cause a clot that will block the coronary artery, resulting in a heart attack.

People with this kind of angina experience chest pain that is predictable, both in onset and intensity. Stable angina can be managed with cardiac medications, especially nitroglycerin, a drug that temporarily widens coronary arteries, lowering blood pressure and relieving the need for the heart to work so hard. The vessels then can relax and the pain is relieved.

Unstable angina is the more dangerous form. Like stable angina, chest pain from unstable angina is caused by plaque that forms within the walls of the coronary arteries. Unlike stable angina, though, this plaque is newly formed and soft; it can blister or bubble, and is more likely to rupture.

If a rupture occurs, platelets — the tiny blood cells that trigger clotting — rush to the site to repair it. This collection of cells forms a clot, which can block the artery and result in a heart attack.

Coronary artery disease is a progressive disease, which means that new formations of plaque can occur over hardened ones; in this way, stable angina can become transformed into unstable angina.

Even if you have stable angina, it is still possible that a piece of plaque may break off, causing a clot. So, if you are experiencing angina that is new, or of a stronger intensity than usual, or it is not relieved by nitroglycerin, call 911 and get to the hospital.

Syndrome X: Narrowing of Tiny Vessels

Stable angina and unstable angina are the two most common types. But there is a third, rare type of cardiac chest pain that is known as "microvascular angina," or "Syndrome X."

As I noted earlier, the heart receives most of its blood from the three main coronary arteries, which are located on the heart's surface. However, the heart also has a "microcirculatory" system, which is a network of tiny blood vessels that branch out from the large coronary vessels. These provide oxygen to each of the millions of cells that make up your heart.

If these tiny vessels become narrowed, or if they spasm, they can cause angina-like chest pain. This type of angina occurs more commonly in people with diabetes and women who have gone through menopause. Microvascular angina is generally treated with the same drugs used to manage angina.

Almost all people experience some kind of chest pain at one time or another. Usually, the pain has nothing to do with the heart. This is why I call chest pain "The Great Pretender."

We feel pain when signals are transported to our brain via a complex system of nerves. But these nerves are situated very close together, and the signals can get crossed, much like the wires on an old switchboard.

Oftentimes, we don't feel pain directly from the part of our body that is affected. The result is that pain that seems to be emanating from our heart is actually originating elsewhere in the body.

Here's a rundown on the conditions that cause pain that is commonly mistaken for cardiac pain:

Pulmonary Embolism and Pericarditis

Besides coronary artery disease, there are other types of chest pain that, while not directly related to a heart attack, can represent symptoms of a life-threatening condition.

A pulmonary embolism (PE) is the condition in which a blood clot lodges in the lungs. People at risk for these types of blood clots are those who are obese, inactive, have been recently hospitalized, or have undergone orthopedic surgeries, such as knee or hip replacement.

In addition, travelers seated on long airplane flights are especially vulnerable. A pulmonary embolism is an emergency that requires immediate medical care. Consider taking one or two aspirin before your next plane flight to thin the blood for your trip to prevent a PE.

Another potentially dangerous condition that can cause chest pain is pericarditis, which is an inflammation of the pericardium, the delicate sac that surrounds the heart. This is usually caused by a viral infection, but it can also occur following a heart attack, open-heart surgery, or sometimes for no specific reason.

Pericarditis is treated with anti-inflammatory drugs, or in some cases steroids. If untreated, pericarditis can become very serious.

Acid Reflux

Esophageal dysfunction, which is also known as gastric reflux or GERD (gastroesophageal reflux disease), causes a type of heartburn that is easily mistaken for chest pain. With GERD, stomach acid backs up into the esophagus, stimulating the nerve fibers and causing a burning sensation.

Sometimes this pain (commonly called heartburn) feels like cardiac pain: sharp pain mixed with pressure, occurring in the mid-chest. GERD can affect anyone, but happens more often in people who are overweight. It also may occur after meals, while lying down, or when you first wake up.

If you think you have GERD, see your doctor. There are medications that treat it, such as Histamine-2 (H-2) blockers or Proton Pump Inhibitors (PPI), which are both drugs that block the production of stomach acid. Left untreated, this condition can cause cellular changes in the lining of the esophagus that are a precursor to cancer.

Arthritis

Although arthritis is usually spoken of as a single ailment, the term actually refers to about 100 different forms of the condition. Of those, two specific types can cause cardiac-like pain: osteoarthritis and rheumatoid arthritis.

Osteoarthritis, known also as "wear-and-tear" arthritis, is a joint disease that causes the top layer of cartilage — the tissue covering the bone — to break down and wear away.

When this occurs in the neck, chest, and shoulders, it causes calcium deposits, or "bone spurs" to form. The nerves in these parts of the body are situated next to the ones that carry pain messages from the chest, so pain that emanates from these areas can feel exactly like it's coming from the heart. An X-ray can confirm the diagnosis.

Rheumatoid arthritis (RA) is a chronic disorder that causes inflammation in the small joints of the body, usually the hands and the feet. RA can also cause the lining around the heart to become inflamed, resulting in pain and shortness of breath that mimics angina.

Both these types of arthritis affect women more often than men. In fact, osteoarthritis of the neck commonly causes chest pain in older women. People with RA are at heightened risk for developing coronary artery disease, so their doctor should monitor them closely.

Gallbladder Inflammation

Some time ago, one of my patients came in to the emergency room wracked with agonizing chest pain. Because I knew he had coronary artery disease, I did a cardiac workup on him; however, the test results came back normal.

The mystery was solved when I gave him an ultrasound test for gallbladder disease. The test showed a large collection of gallstones.

Chronic gallbladder disease — inflammation of the gallbladder — can cause acute abdominal pain that radiates to the chest. After the patient's gallbladder was removed, his chest pain disappeared.

Shingles

Shingles, also called herpes zoster, is a condition characterized by skin eruptions on the body. Shingles also causes severe chest pain, and because this symptom can occur before the telltale rash, it is often mistaken for cardiac chest pain.

Shingles is caused by the chicken pox virus, which can remain dormant in the body for years, but then activate due to a weakened immune system. This is a painful, debilitating disease that can cause nerve and muscle damage.

Anyone who has had chicken pox is at risk for developing shingles. Being over 50, having a weakened immune system due to cancer treatment or HIV/AIDS, and taking certain medications that dampen the immune system, like prolonged uses of steroids (prednisone), are added risk factors.

If you are at risk, talk to your doctor about taking a shingles vaccine. It helps prevent the disease, or make it less painful and dangerous.

Inflammation of the Chest Membrane And Rib Joints

Pleurisy is a condition that occurs when the membrane that lines the chest and covers the lungs becomes inflamed. Given its location, it's not surprising that this sharp, localized pain can mimic angina. Unlike angina, however, the pain from pleurisy worsens if you inhale or cough.

Pleurisy can be caused by pneumonia or other lung conditions, including pulmonary hypertension (high blood pressure in the blood vessels carrying blood to the lungs), pulmonary embolus (a blood clot in the lung) or, in some cases, even asthma. It can also be caused by chest trauma, rheumatoid arthritis, or infection.

The treatment for pleurisy depends on the cause. In cases of bacterial infection, antibiotics are used; viral infections will usually clear up on their own. In some cases, surgery may be required to drain fluid.

The rib cage is connected to the breastbone, or sternum, by (costal) cartilage, the bars of hard, rubbery tissue that enable the ribs to flex and move. If these rib joints become inflamed, a painful condition called costochondritis can result.

This type of pain can occur after vigorous exercise or injury, and can be severe enough to suggest heart attack. However, the pain usually resolves with rest. Treatments include painkillers, and in rare cases cortisone injections or surgery.

Sometimes, costochondritis may appear after a respiratory flu-like illness, but this ailment can also occur for no apparent reason.

Anxiety

Anxiety is a common cause of chest pain, particularly in women. However, this can be a hot-button topic because for many years heart disease in women was overlooked, and women were often told that the chest pain was "all in their heads."

We now know better. But this doesn't erase the fact that, sometimes, women do suffer from chest pain that is a manifestation of anxiety or panic attacks. In fact, panic attacks (also known as panic disorder) mimic not only coronary chest pain, but other heart attack symptoms as well, often inducing a pounding heartbeat, dizziness, and a feeling of doom. These symptoms can be so convincing that many patients end up in the emergency room.

If you are a woman with chest pain, make sure your doctor takes your complaint seriously, especially if you have major risk factors for coronary heart disease, such as high blood pressure, high cholesterol, diabetes, or if you smoke.

If your doctor performs a cardiac evaluation and rules out coronary artery disease, consider seeing some type of counselor or therapist who can teach you how to deal with stress. Prayer also is often a powerful stress reducer.

These days, if you arrive at an emergency room complaining of chest pain, an overnight stay most likely will be required. On one hand, this is good because many heart attacks that would have been missed can now be detected. On the other hand, no one wants the expense and inconvenience of an overnight stay and cardiac evaluation if they are suffering chest pain from another cause.

Still, if you are at risk for a heart attack, and experience symptoms that could be a heart attack, call 911 and ask to be taken to the hospital.

If you do not have major risk factors for a heart attack, you may be experiencing one of the other common causes of chest pain. The best thing to do then is call your doctor and make an appointment to be seen as soon as possible.

CHAPTER 9

The Truth About Women and Heart Disease

Here's a fact that might surprise you: Since 1984, more women have died from heart disease than men. In fact, heart disease now is the No. 1 cause of death among American women, surpassing all types of cancer combined. In 2006, heart disease killed 432,709 women in the U.S. (35 percent of all deaths of women), while all types of cancer caused 269,819 deaths of women (22 percent), according to the American Heart Association.

In spite of these alarming statistics, most women don't realize that they are at risk for heart disease. Many continue to believe that heart disease is something that happens only to men.

The source of this misunderstanding is twofold. For one thing, many physicians still don't fully understand or recognize the symptoms of heart disease in women. For another, most women don't know or acknowledge that heart disease can happen to them, despite some recent public health campaigns.

The result of this dynamic of ignorance between physicians and patients is that at-risk women aren't being screened or treated for heart disease correctly. Health problems such as hypertension and high cholesterol aren't diagnosed at an early stage, and can progress to severe disease before women seek medical attention — or, worse yet, end up in the ER.

Women have the same major risk factors for heart disease as men do, including history of smoking, obesity, high cholesterol, inactive lifestyle, and high blood pressure. A family history is also indicative, though it may be harder for women to identify the disease in their forebears, as previous deaths may have been attributed to other causes.

Women generally start presenting with heart disease in their 60s, an average of 10 years later than men. When they do develop the disease, they are twice as likely to have a second heart attack within six years of the first; they have a greater chance of dying from the disease; and they generally have worse outcomes with bypass or stenting procedures.

The 10-year difference in age of presentation with heart disease usually is attributed to the effect of menopause. When women reach menopause, there are a few factors that increase their risk of heart disease. For one thing, as metabolism slows, there is a tendency toward weight gain, primarily in the abdomen and thighs — this is crucial, as a waist circumference of more than 35 inches is considered an important factor for heart disease in women.

Higher cholesterol levels also are common, and spikes in blood pressure are not uncommon. In fact, the rate of hypertension in women, compared with men, increases steadily with age. Hypertension affects more men than women, according to the AHA, before the age of 45. Women and men are affected at about the same rate between the ages of 45 and 64. But after 64, women have higher rates of hypertension than men.

Hormones Influence Heart Disease

The rate of heart disease in women is two to three times greater after they have reached menopause than in women who are the exact same age but have not reached menopause, according to research from the Cleveland Clinic. This points to the fact that estrogen is another key factor in the incidence of heart disease in women.

Both the heart and the arteries contain estrogen receptors. When estrogen is circulating freely in the bloodstream, it binds to these receptors, causing a release of nitric oxide. Nitric oxide is crucial to a healthy cardiovascular system, as it signals the muscles in the arteries to relax, allowing the arteries to dilate and blood flow to increase. This prevents plaque buildup on the artery walls. All of these factors work together to keep hypertension at bay and ensure that the circulatory process works smoothly, and that the heart is not overworked.

The presence of estrogen also tends to increase the levels of HDL cholesterol (the good kind) and decrease the levels of LDL cholesterol (the bad kind). However, that has not translated into a reduction in heart disease and heart attacks when post-menopausal women receive estrogen therapy.

Although recent studies of hormone replacement therapy (HRT) are not 100 percent conclusive about the benefits of hormone replacement for heart disease, it appears to be safe to take a short course in order to relieve common symptoms caused by menopause (hot flashes, vaginal dryness, and insomnia, among others).

HRT also can help raise metabolism, which hinders weight gain, and boost energy levels, allowing for a more active lifestyle. The women I've known who have taken HRT have done well. They appear more youthful, they have a higher metabolic rate and lower levels of cholesterol, and they seem to show a greater sense of overall well-being.

One concern with HRT has been that it results in additional risk of breast and ovarian cancer. Use of bioidentical hormones may minimize that risk.

Although I support the use of HRT as a short-course treatment, it is an option that each woman needs to discuss with her physician, as medical history and present state of health may determine whether or not it is appropriate.

Atypical Disease Symptoms in Women

Just as women have the same basic risk factors related to heart disease in men, their basic symptoms are the same. These include chest pain, pains radiating down the shoulder, arm, or back; shortness of breath; sweating; and nausea or vomiting.

Although men and women have the same classic symptoms, women have a greater rate of atypical symptoms. In fact, one study found that 43 percent of women who experienced a heart attack did not report chest pain.

Unfortunately, atypical symptoms have been either ignored or downplayed as simple health issues that women face every day. These symptoms include indigestion, shortness of breath, sweating, anxiety or confusion, a burning feeling in the chest, fainting, backache, neck ache, and even pain in the jaw.

In the past, these symptoms were often attributed to anxiety, and because of the lack of consideration of these symptoms as serious problems, many women shrugged them off as inconveniences and did not seek treatment.

Women also need to speak to their doctors in the plainest terms possible. Women have a greater tendency than men to interpret their symptoms rather than simply describing them. By claiming they have a stomach ache that nausea is causing, women might get that diagnosis back, instead of letting the physician ask all the necessary questions to get a proper diagnosis.

Because of this history, women tend to postpone treatment even today— they are less likely to believe they are having a heart attack and wait before going to an ER or calling an ambulance. This needs to change to ensure that women receive the best care possible to help their recovery.

Other risk factors women need to be aware of include the presence of chronic inflammatory disease and pregnancy-induced conditions such as pre-eclampsia and hypertension.

The presence of chronic systemic inflammation, which is more common in women than in men, may facilitate the depositing of plaque on artery walls, according to the *Harvard Health Letter*. Women are also more likely to have chronic inflammatory conditions such as lupus, which doubles the risk of having a heart attack.

During pregnancy, a woman's body goes through many changes, including hormone fluctuations, water retention, and weight gain — all of which are considered normal. Some women, however, also experience conditions that can become red flags for future heart disease.

Pregnancy-induced hypertension, pre-eclampsia (a condition that includes hypertension and protein in the urine), and gestational diabetes (in which the body becomes insulin-resistant) are all potential problems that can arise from pregnancy. Up to 10 percent of pregnant women experience pregnancy-induced hypertension, and up to 7 percent of pregnancies experience gestational diabetes — though recent research indicates that number is increasing.

Most women return to their normal health state postpartum. However, the fact that these conditions appeared at all is an indication that a woman has a predisposition for heart disease and/or diabetes. Women who have experienced gestational diabetes have a 60 percent chance of developing Type 2 diabetes later in life, according to the Cleveland Clinic. And women who experienced severe preeclampsia during pregnancy have a 60 percent greater risk for heart disease later in life.

At face value, that may seem like bad news. But it can have a positive outcome because women who suffer through those conditions during pregnancy know at a relatively young age that they are at risk.

And knowing is half the battle. They can change their lifestyles and be proactive in seeking baseline testing in order to minimize the chance for hypertension, heart disease, and diabetes later in life.

Traditional Perspective Is Changing

In the past, women ran the household and men paid the bills and took care of financial matters. Women were perceived, from a historical and sociological perspective, to be under less stress than men.

As a result, heart disease historically has been considered a "man's disease." Even when women did show symptoms, these were shrugged off as emotional anxiety or attributed to some other cause. When it came to heart disease, physicians based their treatments on information that came from studies focused specifically on the male population.

Today, all that has changed.

More than ever before, women are facing the same workplace stresses that men face. What's more, in dual-income homes, women still carry a greater share of responsibility, which translates into more stress as the primary homemakers and caretakers. This contributes to the trend of heart disease occurring more frequently among working women. One study indicated that these women have a 40 percent greater risk of heart disease.

In addition, as women spend more time at work, they pick up the bad habits of careerism, particularly the tendency to eat out, which undeniably leads to unhealthy eating habits.

When taking all these circumstances into account, it is imperative that women begin to realize they are at increased risk for heart disease.

In general, heart disease treatments for women are identical to those for men: weight reduction, healthier eating habits, exercise, elimination of smoking, reduction of stress, and medications and supplements as needed. This includes statins and ACE inhibitors (to treat hypertension) on a limited-time basis.

If women are not diabetic, don't smoke, and do not have high blood pressure, they should see their primary care physician for baseline testing of cholesterol in their 40s. About 10 years after menopause, they should have a stress test and EKG.

I also recommend one teaspoon of cod liver oil daily for women. This provides vitamin D, which helps reduce blood pressure and has been proven to reduce risk of heart disease. Premenopausal women with a vitamin D deficiency have three times greater risk of developing systolic hypertension within 15 years than women with normal vitamin D levels.

I do worry about the smokers and the diabetics, who face an accelerated disease state. These patients also tend to present later, and have more severe disease as more arteries are involved and are extremely narrowed.

Follow-up is crucial for every patient, but even more so for women with heart disease. Because they tend to present later in life, they are likely to have other medical conditions that could complicate treatment and affect their health.

Because of their anatomies, women also tend to have a quicker relapse rate than men, which means that monitoring heart health is imperative so treatment or interventions can be modified or implemented on an immediate basis when needed.

Reversing History

As I noted, in past generations most women didn't know if there was a history of heart disease for female members of their family because that data was not tracked. Luckily, that data is now being collected.

Yet even without this data, there are changes that can be made to anyone's lifestyle that can reduce predisposition toward disease. We all have genetic tendencies, but we also have the ability to turn off that "genetic switch."

By eating healthy, exercising, avoiding smoking, and limiting other risk factors as much as we can, we can significantly reduce our chances of having heart disease. By getting treatment when we recognize a problem — rather than waiting until the problem gets serious — we can improve our outcomes.

Women need to seek baseline testing, make lifestyle modifications, and seek immediate medical treatment if they feel they are having heart problems. Don't brush off the symptoms as mere anxiety. Listen to what your body is telling you.

The bottom line is that women present at an older age, with more advanced disease, and have worse outcomes than men. It's not a combination for good health or one that is particularly reassuring. But the information needed to understand the risk, symptoms, and how to help minimize risk factors is out there, as are the public health campaigns to educate both women and physicians.

Pay attention, and get your physician to pay attention, too. Your health depends on it.

PART TWO

Treat It!

CHAPTER 10

Must-Have Heart Tests

Our ability to determine whether someone is at risk for heart disease has improved significantly during the past 30 years.

Although no single test can tell the whole story of a person's risk for heart disease, part of the story can be gained through long-standing tools, and the information these tools provide actually means more today because of our advanced understanding of heart disease.

Then again, because of what these sophisticated measurements tell us, additional risk factors are coming into view only now.

Anyone at risk for heart disease — and that means almost everyone over 50 — should know about the "Fabulous 15" tests that help your doctor assess your heart health. In fact, a couple of these are so new that your doctor may not even know about them, or may not yet be in the habit of using them regularly.

You may have undergone a number of these tests and wondered what the technician was looking for, or how the data might help your doctor. It's far better that patients understand these things personally — because if you do, you'll have a much better chance of changing the behaviors that are having a negative impact on your health.

The Fabulous 15 Heart Tests

1. Ultrasound of the Carotid Arteries. This is one of the new studies providing a lot of helpful information. The carotids are large arteries in the neck, close to the surface, that supply blood to the brain. Ultrasound is totally noninvasive. The patient does nothing but lie still while the ultrasound monitor passes over his neck. Using this method, we can measure plaque buildup in the arteries.

Baseline studies have established how thick the carotid arteries should be, specifically the inner layer — called the intima — of the arteries. Significant thickening in the carotid arteries signals heart disease, and the degree of thickening tells us how severe this heart disease is — not only in the carotids but also throughout the cardiovascular system. Studies can even reveal the "age" of the arteries, showing that a 40-year-old man might have the carotid arteries of an 80-year-old.

Regression of heart disease shows up in these tests as well. Indeed, ultrasound is one of the best ways of showing patients that the measures they are taking to control their heart disease are paying off. The test takes only 15 minutes for a technician to perform at a qualified cardiologist's office.

2. Blood Pressure Screening. This is a common test that most people have had. A person can have elevated blood pressure and feel nothing out of the ordinary. The elderly benefit through having low blood pressure, with decreased incidence of stroke, heart attack, myocardial infarction, and organ damage, such as to the eyes or kidneys.

A good blood pressure reading is around 120/80. Specifically, it should be less than 140/90. Both the top measure (systolic) and the bottom measure (diastolic) are important. Historically, doctors tended to discount the systolic because that number tends to creep up as we age. However, in recent years, we've found that this measure also needs to stay low for all age groups.

3. C-Reactive Protein Test. This test reports inflammatory changes in the body. Elevated inflammation puts us at increased risk for heart attacks. General inflammation can be treated simply with aspirin and statin drugs.

Inflammation used to be regarded as a "marker" of heart disease, meaning that it is seen in patients who already have heart disease. The latest studies indicate, however, that inflammation is actually a driver of heart disease.

4. Lipid Panel. Most of us are familiar with blood tests for cholesterol. Make sure that your doctor includes a lipid panel — a set of tests indicating the various types of fat in the blood — in your next screening.

A lipid panel offers a pattern of your LDL cholesterol, which sometimes is called "bad" cholesterol. But not all LDL cholesterol is created equal. The smaller and denser your LDL particles are, the more dangerous they are. These new pattern studies indicate whether a patient's LDL cholesterol fits into Pattern A, meaning the particles are large and less dense; or Pattern B, meaning smaller and denser. Pattern B is a warning sign.

Small, dense LDL particles are more likely to embed in the arterial wall. This starts the heart disease chain reaction. An embedded fat particle attracts other fat particles, creating plaque buildup. The body tries to cure this condition by sealing the plaque with red blood cells, creating something like an internal scab. But this sealing process can get out of control, causing blood clots to form. The rupture of these clots causes most heart attacks and strokes.

Pattern B LDL can be "plumped up" and made less destructive through taking vitamin B-3 (niacin). Omega-3 fish oils also can be helpful in changing the character of these particles, but not nearly as much as niacin.

5. Diabetic Screening. Along with a hemoglobin A1C test, you should take a fasting blood sugar test. Your fasting blood sugar level should be less than 100; any number greater than that indicates either a problem with metabolic syndrome, or pre-diabetes or full-blown Type 2 (late onset) diabetes.

Many foolish people try to outwit the fasting test by changing their eating habits a couple of days before the test. That's why I advocate the hemoglobin A1C test, which provides a retrospective picture of a person's glucose level during the past three months. It can't be outwitted.

If the reading on the hemoglobin A1C test is greater than 6, that means the patient's blood sugar has been unacceptably high during the past three months, no matter what their fasting blood sugar count may be.

6. Step on the Scale! The most important piece of "exercise equipment" in the home is the humble scale. Many people put off weighing themselves, thinking that they'll do it after they start to exercise more or improve their diet. Don't wait! Weigh yourself now, and do it every day.

Diet and exercise programs typically advise people to weigh themselves less frequently, assuming that small, naturally occurring fluctuations of 1 or 2 pounds will be frustrating. But if you don't weigh yourself every day, you easily can get out of the habit, and before you know it that extra 5 pounds becomes 10, then 20. Vacation and holiday eating will add pound after pound if you blind yourself to their effects. Weighing yourself promptly after Thanksgiving weekend or after that summer cruise will help you reduce your caloric intake in the following week.

As we get older, we lose muscle mass because of decreasing testosterone and estrogen levels. This results in excess calories being stored as fat rather than being burned off. With that, a self-perpetuating process begins: As we gain weight, our appetite for fatty foods and carbohydrates increases, resulting in additional weight. Worse yet, weight gain encourages a sedentary lifestyle — and that leads to even more weight gain.

Everyone should have a body mass index (BMI) of less than 25. That means no more than 25 percent of your total body weight is attributable to fat. If your BMI is over 25, the fats and sugar in your blood are likely to skyrocket. Most people should remain about what they weighed at graduation from high school or college. You need to track your progress toward or away from that target daily.

7. Abdominal Aortic Aneurysm Screening. I recommend this test, conducted via ultrasound of the abdomen, for anyone over 50. If you are 65 or older, Medicare will pay for it if you have any smoking history.

Smoking only 100 cigarettes in your life puts you at risk for abdominal aortic aneurysm. The aorta runs behind the navel. This test looks for an aorta diameter of less than 3 centimeters. If it's larger than that, an aneurysm (abnormal widening or ballooning of a portion of an artery because of weakness in the wall of the blood vessel) is developing. Aneurysms can rupture, leading to internal bleeding and other serious consequences.

The noninvasive ultrasound test for aortic aneurysm can be done in just 5 to 10 minutes. An aortic aneurysm can be treated easily with cholesterol reduction, blood pressure control, and diabetic control.

8. PLAC Test. This new study, performed through blood screening, evaluates the likelihood of plaque rupturing within vessels. Its predictive value is coming into focus only now, but the test seems to be remarkably accurate in identifying the primary initiator of most heart attacks and strokes.

9. Check Hormone Levels. Because of the drop in testosterone and estrogen levels in men and women over 50, it's a good idea to have your hormone levels checked.

In men, low testosterone leads to loss of muscle mass, weight gain, poor sexual performance, depression, and elevated cholesterol. In middle age, men go through their own form of menopause — or, as it's sometimes called, "male pause" or "man-o-pause." Testosterone levels can be checked through a simple blood test, though interpreting the results is not so simple.

Because so few of us had our testosterone levels checked before middle age, the "normal" spectrum is wide — from 280 to 800 ng/dl. Some men feel normal at the low end of this range, while others do not.

Hormone replacement therapy (usually in the form of testosterone creams and injections) is indicated for men whose testosterone falls below 280. It also may be indicated for those above this lower threshold because every man's "normal" is different. Work with your doctor to get the counts in a range that brings improvement in vitality and cholesterol levels.

Recent articles indicate that there may be some risk attached to hormone replacement therapy, particularly with regard to exacerbating the growth of undetected prostate cancer. Make sure to discuss these risks with your physician.

10. Thyroid Levels. It's also important to check your thyroid function. If thyroid levels are too low (hypothyroidism), your cholesterol levels are likely to climb, and you could become sugar intolerant.

11. Ankle-Brachial Index. This test can help detect and measure peripheral artery disease (PAD), which results in pain in the legs while exercising, and is a sure sign of cardiovascular disease.

To detect the presence of PAD, a patient's blood pressure is taken with one cuff on the upper arm and one at the ankle. The two measurements should be nearly the same. If the two differ significantly, this indicates PAD — the presence of a blockage in the aorta or in the legs.

12. Echocardiogram. This test uses an ultrasound device placed between the ribs of the left chest to create a picture of the whole heart. The test evaluates how well the chambers of the heart are pumping or contracting, as well as measuring the dimensions of the four chambers of the heart. This gives an indication of whether the heart is of normal size or dilated.

The test also measures the thickness of the heart muscle, which aids in the detection of high blood pressure.

An echocardiogram enables doctors to take a look at all four valves of the heart. These can be damaged because of rheumatic fever, or may show degenerative changes that are the result of aging. These changes can lead to heart murmurs, which cause the heart to work harder to pump the same amount of blood.

This is one of the best tests doctors have to assess the heart at rest. It reveals the heart's "ejection fraction": the amount of blood the heart ejects with every beat, which should be 55 percent or more. Underlying heart disease often shows up in a reduced ejection fraction.

People with an ejection fraction of 35 to 55 percent can lead a productive life with the help of medication. Below 35 percent, people are at risk for sudden death. They should have a defibrillator installed surgically.

13. EKG (electrocardiogram). This test gives doctors the ability to look at the heart through 12 different windows, each identifying a particular area of the heart. Most patients have a normal EKG the first time it's administered. With good record-keeping, this allows us to detect changes in the heart over time. Such changes are one of the easiest ways to know when further tests are warranted.

An EKG is based on the way electrical current travels through the heart. Usually, the current travels on a diagonal from the right shoulder down to the left leg. If someone has had a heart attack or damage to the heart, the direction of the electrical impulse changes, usually in the region where the damage has occurred.

Think of the 12 different windows of the EKG as so many kites in the wind. All the kites should be flying in the same direction. If 11 kites are flying in one direction, and one kite is flying in another direction, we know something is wrong. The way this shows up on the readout is that the angle of the electrical wave is altered wherever the problem is.

14. Stress Test. This is probably the most well-known heart study. We've all seen pictures of people walking on treadmills with electrodes attached to their chests. A stress test is often administered after the identification of a problem, but it can be a good screening tool as well.

Everyone should have a stress test after the age of 50. This opinion has become somewhat controversial, but as a cardiologist, I know that there's a high incidence of cardiac problems in people who previously have shown no evidence of heart disease. Several factors taken together put a huge percentage of the population at risk: 50 percent of the population is overweight, many are smokers or were in the past, and family history or genetic inheritance plays a role as well.

There are different kinds of stress tests. The most basic is walking on a treadmill where the incline and speed are adjusted every three minutes. Most people can last on the treadmill between seven and 10 minutes — few go over 10 minutes.

While the person walks on the treadmill, doctors evaluate the EKG, the test subject's blood pressure, pulse rate, and color and demeanor. It's important to be aware of the whole person, such as whether the patient looks anxious or grows ashen, because these are warning signs no matter what the EKG says.

False positives and false negatives go with this basic form of stress test, so other forms of the study have been developed. One is called the nuclear cardiology stress test, in which the subject walks on the treadmill again, but is then injected with a nuclear isotope at the end of the exercise. This isotope settles in the heart muscle, and we can take pictures of the heart with a nuclear camera.

In these pictures, the heart lights up like a lantern wherever there's good blood profusion. If an area of the heart remains dark, we know that blood isn't flowing as it should.

Another stress test is called the stress echo study. Again, the study begins with the patient walking on a treadmill as his EKG, blood pressure, and pulse rate are monitored. We take an echocardiogram at rest to get a baseline of how the heart is doing; we take another at the peak of exercise; and then we overlay the images to see if there's any defect or dropout or decreased contraction. If there is, that usually indicates a blockage.

The downside to this test is that it has the tendency to miss patients who have single-vessel disease — that is, disease in only one artery. In those cases, the other arteries compensate for the disease in the one vessel, and a doctor can't pick it up on the echocardiogram.

The stress test — even in its simplest form — does have a powerful predictive value. If a patient can stay on the treadmill for 10 minutes or longer with the standard protocol, the incidence of a cardiac event — such as heart attack or stroke — during the next 12 months is near zero, even if that patient has heart disease.

The risks associated with a stress test are fewer than people imagine. I've been performing such tests for more than 30 years and never have lost a patient. But make sure you are working with qualified physicians and personnel.

One last word of warning: Passing a stress test doesn't mean that no heart disease is present — it indicates only that the patient is doing reasonably well. If a patient continues to have symptoms, he or she needs to be evaluated further.

15. CT Scans. This test now is being used in certain instances to screen for coronary artery disease. Unfortunately, it's not very accurate if you already have advanced heart disease with lots of calcification. These calcium deposits cast shadows that can be read falsely as blockages. Anyone who has a high calcium count in the arteries should probably avoid having a CT scan.

In addition, a CT scan delivers a high dose of radiation — the equivalent of 400 chest X-rays. For this reason, the use of CT scans as a diagnostic tool for heart disease is falling out of favor with doctors. There's evidence that 10 years after the test, some people who have had CT scans suffer a higher incidence of leukemia and lymphoma.

Heart catheterization, in which a plastic tube (catheter) is inserted in an artery in the leg and threaded into the heart, delivers a far lower dose of radiation and gives a complete picture of what's happening in the major arteries and the heart.

I advise patients who are considering a CT scan to get a catheterization instead. Not only do we get more accurate information, but also, if blockages are detected, we can implant stents that usually restore normal circulation immediately.

CHAPTER 11

7 Steps for Living Statin-Free

Statin medications are highly controversial. They are the most widely prescribed drugs in the United States and their potential side effects have become a hot issue. As our understanding of the heart disease story continues to evolve, some have questioned the role statins play in reducing heart disease.

I advise my patients to see statins, whenever possible, as an interventional medication rather than an excuse to keep living an unhealthy lifestyle. It's my goal to educate my patients and to help them transition to a lifestyle that makes statins unnecessary. (Because of genetic factors, this is not always possible.) Living statin-free presents challenges, of course, but it can be done.

There are two things that every person taking a statin medication needs to know:

• The reasons for taking a statin medication.
• How these medications can be left behind.

I want patients with no known underlying heart disease to have a total cholesterol count under 200. Those with previously diagnosed heart disease need to have a count under 150.

With patients who have not had a cardiac event or a stroke, I wait for two to three months before prescribing a statin, first asking the patient to change his or her lifestyle. If a patient cannot achieve these goals after the monitoring period, I then prescribe a statin medication.

What Are Statins and What Do They Do?
Despite what the fear-mongers say, your doctor is not in cahoots with the pharmaceutical companies to drain your wallet. The bottom line is that statins work. In the past 10 years there has been a 27 percent reduction in fatal heart attacks, and much of this improvement is due to statins.

Statins block an enzyme in the liver called hydroxy-methylglu-taryl-coenzyme A (HMG-CoA) reductase, which is responsible for producing cholesterol. These drugs are particularly effective at reducing LDL cholesterol, lowering counts by 25 percent to 55 percent.

The newer statins, mildly raise the "good cholesterol" HDL by 5 percent to 15 percent. They also reduce another form of fat in the blood, triglycerides, by 10 percent to 25 percent.

But that's not all statins do. They are also vasodilators — they help expand or widen arteries, increasing blood flow during exercise.

Statins also improve the function of the endothelial cells that line the arteries. This is particularly important because we know that damage to the arterial lining starts the process of plaque formation. It's the rupturing of plaque deposits that leads to the blood clots responsible for most heart attacks.

Statins help maintain plaque stability, preventing the plaque deposits that have already formed from rupturing. By both protecting endothelial cells and maintaining plaque stability, statins help prevent blood clots.

Statins Reduce Your Risk of Heart Disease, Period

Statins also reduce inflammation in the arteries, which can be seen through blood studies of C-reactive protein.

Indeed, the recent Jupiter Study on men with no other risk factors other than elevated levels of inflammation throughout the body (elevated C-reactive protein) found that statins cut the incidence of heart attack by 54 percent and stroke by 48 percent. The study concluded early because, given these results, it would have been unethical to continue administering placebos to the control group.

Although the "lipid theory" as to the cause of cardiovascular disease — that it's caused by excess fat in the blood — is now widely accepted, doubters remain.

But even the doubters have to acknowledge that statins reduce cardiovascular disease. Whether through their cholesterol-reducing properties, their protective effect on arterial cells, or their anti-inflammatory benefits, the role of statins in curbing heart disease is impressive.

So why then are so many people leery of statins, and why do I try to bridge my patients to a statin-free lifestyle?

The risks associated with statins are real, if grossly exaggerated. There are two chief concerns with statins: liver and muscle damage.

As statins work in the liver, tests show they can sometimes raise the level of liver function. Liver function is usually measured by testing two enzymes, AST (aspartate transaminase) and ALT (alanine transaminase). These indicate inflammation and cell destruction within the liver. If a patient's liver function levels are elevated, that indicates that the statin medication may have introduced some toxicity.

The liver is a big organ and has amazing powers of regeneration. Even cirrhosis of the liver can now be controlled or even reversed if caught in its early stages.

There's no reason to worry about liver damage from statins, however, unless liver function rises to two-and-a-half to three times its normal value. Even when a statin introduces this level of toxicity, taking the patient off a statin medication allows liver function to return to normal.

Every statin is metabolized in the system in a slightly different way. Many cases of elevated liver function tests are statin-specific. Simvastatin might cause elevated liver function in a particular patient while atorvastatin does not — and vice versa. I've rarely had a case where I could not find a statin medication that the patient didn't tolerate well.

I also employ the strategy, based on studies conducted in Europe, of having my patients take their statin drug every other day or every third day. Many patients on this regimen are doing well; their cholesterol counts remain at target.

Liver damage associated with a statin is extremely rare. Usually, such cases involve a history of underlying liver damage that makes the liver vulnerable. This includes conditions like cirrhosis, hepatitis, and iron-overload diseases such as hemochromatosis. Even in these cases, if the doctor is properly monitoring the patient, long-term damage can usually be avoided.

So, I say that if you see your doctor and your liver is reasonably healthy, you have little cause for concern about liver damage from taking a statin.

The other major concern with statins is muscle wasting. Mild forms of this condition are called myopathy. Your doctor can verify whether you are suffering from myopathy by checking your CPK enzymes.

Myopathy causes muscle aches and weakness that can be accompanied by fatigue. The onset of myopathy usually occurs from two weeks to two months after initiating stain treatment. That's why I advise my patients that if they experience any muscle weakness to see me immediately. Even if you just feel unusually listless or fatigued you should have another consultation with your doctor.

A serious form of muscle wasting that can result is called rhabdomyolysis. I cannot stress enough how rare such a development is, but I would not be giving you the whole picture if I did not mention it.

With rhabdomyolysis, muscle breakdown is rapid and the resulting pain can feel like getting hit in the calf with a fastball. Dead muscle cells flood into the bloodstream and can overwhelm the kidneys, resulting in long-term complications.

In a study for the *Journal of the American Medical Association* conducted in 2004, the most popular statins at the time — atorvastatin, pravastatin, and simvastatin — caused one case of rhabdomyolysis for every 22,727 people treated. Death occurred in 1 patient out of a population of 252,460. I have seen only one patient with this condition in more than 25 years of practicing medicine.

Consider these statistics in the context of our heart disease pandemic: Every day, nearly 2,600 Americans die of some type of cardiovascular disease. That's an average of one death every 34 seconds, and 7.1 million Americans have had a heart attack during their lifetimes. You can see why your doctor might prescribe a statin!

Statins have other, minor side effects. These medications slightly elevate a person's risk for developing late-onset diabetes. A recent study led by Naveed Sattar and published in England's *The Lancet* shows that use of statins increases the risk of developing Type 2 diabetes by 9 percent. But the chance of developing diabetes on an absolute basis as the result of taking a statin is low — a risk far outweighed by a statin's benefits.

Reasons to Be Cautious With Statins

There is some evidence that statins can sap a patient's vitality by binding testosterone and estrogen. Cholesterol is involved in the synthesis of steroids, and thus the production of these hormones. If you start taking a statin and your libido takes a vacation, ask your doctor to test your hormone levels.

Don't be embarrassed about this. These hormones also affect mental acuity, your ability to sleep, emotional well-being, and ability to cope with stress. It's important that your hormones are at the appropriate levels. Fortunately, decreases in these essential hormones can be remedied through medication.

Statins also decrease the body's supply of Coenzyme Q10 (CoQ10), which helps make the heart strong. This side effect can be eliminated with the addition of a simple, over-the-counter supplement of Coenzyme Q10 (200 to 400 mg daily).

There is evidence, mostly anecdotal in nature, that statins can cause memory loss and even amnesia, as well as other cognitive defects such as difficulty concentrating. These problems showed up in the first clinical trials, but so infrequently — in less than one-half of 1 percent — that these symptoms have commanded little attention. I just do not see this in my practice.

So why get off statins? These medications do not supply something the body needs. Instead, they prevent the body from producing too much of a substance that it does need, cholesterol, which plays an important role in cell function.

It's understandable then that we'd prefer to remedy the problem by creating conditions in which the body can make the right amount of cholesterol. But let's look squarely at the challenges we face, and take the superior, strictly natural, approach.

Here are the 7 Steps that will give you the best chance of living statin free.

1. **Start with your doctor.** The first step may surprise you because it's not demanding at all. It's a step, however, that many never take or fail to sustain. Build a relationship with your physician. Review your desire to get off statins and where you stand in regard to heart-healthy targets. Then, in consultation with your doctor, put together a game plan for doing so. As I've said, this will demand lifestyle modification. Without changing the way you live there's no solid justification for getting off your statin medication.

2. **Get serious about food.** Part of this game plan must be eating a plant-based diet. Depending on a patient's particular profile, I recommend either the Dean Ornish heart-reversal diet or the South Beach Diet. If you have known heart disease, the Ornish diet is better because it most effectively cleanses the system of excess fat. The South Beach Diet is usually for those with risk factors but no known heart disease. This diet allows more latitude and can still get a person to the recommended targets.

Although the Ornish diet puts no restriction on calorie intake — mainly because it's hard to consume too many calories eating fruits and vegetables — you'll need to limit your calories on the South Beach Diet or a Mediterranean diet. A typical, unrestricted diet for the average adult contains about 2,400 calories per day. Aim to keep your calorie intake to between 1,500 and 1,800 calories. The lower end is for women; the higher end is for men.

3. **Lose weight for good, starting now.** Get to and maintain your ideal body weight. One way to judge your ideal body weight is via body mass index (BMI). Your BMI represents the percentage of your total body weight that's due to fat. It should be under 25. Many health clubs have simple handheld devices that provide a BMI reading. These also can be purchased at drugstores.

Another way to think about ideal body weight is to remember what you weighed as a senior in high school. How far away are you? At that time your total cholesterol count — unless you already had a weight problem — was probably in the 120s. That's the range that's typical in populations without heart disease. So think "high school skinny." For many of us, that's a long way to go. You'll need to approach this target weight, though, to sufficiently change your biochemistry.

1. **Get moving on a daily basis.** Start exercising five days a week for one hour per day. Walking is generally the best exercise available because it doesn't place too much stress on the knees, hips, and back. If you like to run, you may want to mix running into your walks, which is how people have been moving ever since civilization began. Tennis and ballroom dancing are good. The invention of golf carts decreased the health value of that sport appreciably. But you can swim or ride a bike.

2. **Shut-eye can save your life.** You must get plenty of sleep — much more than our workaholic culture commonly believes. Not just eight hours a night, but eight to 10 hours on a regular basis. Sleep is the body's main way of dealing with stress. Specifically, and this might surprise you, lack of sleep results in the liver pumping out excess cholesterol!

3. **Change your perspective on life.** Besides sleeping more, it's important to take additional measures to reduce stress. The

greatest of these is recruiting the support of your loved ones. Talk to your wife, husband, or others in your life about your desire to live in a healthy way. Rely on them for the encouragement and accountability you need.

4. **Slash your cholesterol counts.** Remember, there are only two ways to reduce your cholesterol: Stop the production of cholesterol in your liver, or stop its absorption in the small intestine.

Adding supplements to your diet can help reduce cholesterol, but most people have to be at their targets, eating right, and exercising before supplements can help them stay there.

One supplement works through the liver just like a statin — because it is a statin, a natural one. Mevastatin is produced naturally by red rice yeast. You can add red rice yeast to your diet by picking up a container at the grocery or health foods store.

Be careful of the provider, however. In the past couple of years there have been problems with red rice yeast produced in China. Suppliers were adding pravastatin to their product to heighten its cholesterol-reducing properties. This posed a health risk as the amount of statin people were taking — unknowingly — varied wildly.

Omega-3 fatty acids from fish oil and vitamin B3 (niacin), remain the champions of the supplements. Both fish oil and niacin boost HDL, plump up LDL particles, and reduce inflammation. Fish oil even has a mild analgesic effect, for which your aching joints will thank you.

New evidence is emerging that flaxseed contains three ingredients that aid in maintaining heart health. Flaxseed is rich with the plant form of omega-3 fatty acids, lignans, which contain both plant estrogen and antioxidant qualities, plus soluble and insoluble fiber. Flaxseed seems to help not only with a person's cholesterol profile but even in maintaining heart rhythm.

Organic grape juice, apples, and other foods that contain pectin help eliminate cholesterol through the gut. Garlic has a mild effect as well.

For those with risk factors or established heart disease, the challenges of living statin free in our culture can be daunting. If you take the seven steps I've outlined, though, starting with establishing that all-important relationship with your physician, you'll have the best chance of success. You'll feel 1,000 times better, too — that I can promise.

CHAPTER 12

8 Steps to Reducing High Blood Pressure

Hypertension, or high blood pressure, may be the medical condition patients deny most frequently. Everyone wants to believe that he or she only suffers from "white coat syndrome" — that is, that their blood pressure is perfect except in the doctor's office. "The worry makes the reading high!" a typical patient protests. "Otherwise, I'm just fine."

Doctors used to think the same thing and would pay little attention to slightly elevated blood pressure readings. Now we've found that "white coat syndrome" is in fact highly predictive of long-term problems with hypertension.

Once I was among those who denied my own hypertension. My readings were normal or only slightly elevated during my checkups. I had reason to suspect, though, that during my stressful workdays my blood pressure was anything but normal. Still, I let my hypertension go for years without treatment.

The trouble is, a single, isolated reading is an insufficient gauge of a person's blood pressure. I should have taken the time to keep a blood pressure diary over a two-week period, taking readings morning and night and at odd times as well. That's the best way to know whether there's a problem with hypertension.

High blood pressure is called "the silent killer" for a reason. Yet, I'm afraid that the tag is so well-known that people don't take it seriously anymore. The first step to lowering high blood pressure is to understand its nature and its devastating effects on your health, and particularly its role in cardiovascular and kidney disease.

To understand the basic phenomenon of blood pressure, think of a garden hose. When water flows through a hose unimpeded, the pressure in the hose is normal — it's strong enough and flexible enough to handle the force of the water.

The amount of pressure the water exerts equals flow times resistance. Step on the hose and you increase the resistance, so the hose has to expand to accommodate the pressure.

Keep forcing the water through the hose without lifting your foot and the hose will eventually explode, ballooning and then rupturing at its weakest point. These same principles operate within your body.

The underlying cause of most high blood pressure — what's known as "essential hypertension" — is a mystery. (Paradoxically, we know that the same conditions that produce hypertension in some people have little or no effect in others.) We know volumes, however, about what makes hypertension worse and how it combines with other factors to produce heart and kidney disease.

Aside from essential hypertension, the causes of "secondary hypertension" are well-known, too. These include obstructive sleep apnea, Cushing's syndrome, congenital obstruction of the aorta, and endocrine disorders such as hyper- and hypothyroidism. Cases where a specific cause can be detected account for about 10 percent of all diagnoses.

It may surprise you to know that the body's main controllers of blood pressure are the kidneys. These two bean-shaped organs are located in your lower back, underneath the rib cage. Together, they filter approximately 200 quarts of blood a day, removing about two quarts of water and waste materials. The water and waste are made into urine and sent to the bladder for excretion.

Your Kidneys and Your Heart

Waste removal takes place in the kidneys in structures called nephrons. Each nephron has an ingenious filtering mechanism called a glomerulus, a specially designed blood vessel or capillary connected to a urine-collecting tubule. The glomerulus keeps normal proteins and cells in the bloodstream while directing extra fluids and wastes to the tubule.

Each nephron also features a network of tiny blood vessels — arterioles — that wrap around the tubule. These networks carry blood that must be filtered to the nephron and then carry the clean, healthy blood away. The kidneys also regulate the level of chemicals such as sodium (salt), phosphorus, and potassium that are released back into the body; they maintain the body's balance of these essential substances.

The kidneys also secrete three important hormones: erythropoietin (EPO), which stimulates the bone marrow to make red blood cells; a regulator of blood pressure called rennin; and calcitriol, the active form of Vitamin D, which helps maintain bone strength.

Researchers have speculated that not all kidneys are created equal. It may be that those whose blood pressure continues to be normal throughout life are blessed with a greater number of, more efficient, or simply hardier glomeruli than others. When a sufficient number of glomeruli are no longer operating, the still-healthy glomeruli send a signal to the system to increase blood pressure so that the remaining vessels can perform the necessary filtering.

The mysterious nature of essential hypertension has led to speculation that there may be a genetic basis for the disease. We don't understand the complexities of the picture yet. But a genetic basis is hard to doubt because ethnicity correlates with rates of high blood pressure.

According to the American Heart Association, more than 40 percent of African Americans suffer from high blood pressure while about 30 percent of non-Hispanic whites do. Hypertension also presents much earlier in African Americans and is often more severe. High blood pressure, like heart disease, also runs in families.

The heart and the arteries are living organisms. They respond to increases in pressure in a more complex and adaptable way than a garden hose. All of the body's arteries can dilate (expand) or constrict (narrow) in response to the body's needs.

In a healthy person, exercise causes the arteries to dilate as the heart beats more rapidly and blood flow increases dramatically. At the end of a good workout, the blood vessels return to normal.

Chronic high blood pressure causes the arteries to inflate like a balloon that's blown up to near-bursting over and over again. When deflated, the balloon bears stretch marks where its structural integrity has been weakened. Once this damage occurs, the balloon loses some of its elasticity. It becomes much easier to blow up and prone to bursting.

The same thing happens with our arteries. When dilated too often by high blood pressure, arteries begin to lose their elasticity and undergo structural damage. Small gaps open between cell junctions as the arterial wall experiences micro-tears. Low-density lipoprotein (LDL) cholesterol particles begin to embed in these crevices, forming waxy plaque deposits.

Over time, the plaque formation calcifies and becomes fibrotic. This restores strength to the arterial wall but at the price of flexibility. The more this process occurs, the less elastic the arteries become, causing atherosclerosis (hardening of the arteries).

At the same time, the artery narrows. Once a major coronary artery narrows more than 50 percent, the heart must beat harder and more rapidly to maintain sufficient blood flow. The original blood pressure problem worsens.

Effects of High Blood Pressure

From this point in the hypertension-induced sequence, several catastrophic problems may follow, as well as minor issues.

If the artery loses 75 percent of its blood-flow capacity, say in an artery of the heart, the person will likely experience pains in the left arm or chest, which is angina. This can be either stable angina, an onset of symptoms that come and go with physical exertion, or unstable angina, a condition that foreshadows a heart attack.

With unstable angina, the attacks "crescendo" or become progressively worse. They can begin suddenly, while the person is at rest, and last more than 15 minutes. Unstable angina demands immediate medical attention.

Cracks may also appear in calcified or partially calcified plaque deposits. Plaque deposits are like evil candy bars with gooey centers. The body tries to heal these cracks by filling them with blood clots, applying a type of scab. These clots ordinarily help with the healing process but at the cost of enlarging the plaque deposit, extending it farther into the artery and reducing blood flow.

Worse yet, the clotting process can go haywire. The clot can keep growing until it ruptures and is released into the bloodstream. The still-soft waxy interior of the original plaque deposit can be released into the bloodstream as well. This biological shrapnel is the usual cause of heart attacks and strokes. It completely blocks one of the major coronary arteries, impairs the function of the heart itself, or travels to the brain from a damaged artery of the neck. With blood flow at a minimum, the tissues begin to die.

Hypertension and excess fat in the blood combine in a degenerative feedback loop — the effects of the original damage to the arteries, however small, make the causes of that damage progressively worse. The cycle begins to repeat.

Even when a heart attack does not occur from hypertension, the heart senses that it has to work harder to maintain blood flow. So its walls will thicken and become stronger in response. As plaque build-up continues, the heart has to work ever harder.

At some point the heart will give up the struggle to become ever stronger and simply dilate and become fatigued, resulting in decreased blood flow. A dilated heart no longer pumps efficiently, though, and this causes the body's other systems to function less efficiently. Water begins to build up in the system as the onset of heart failure begins.

Or, high blood pressure can stress particular areas of the arterial system, even without the presence of plaque deposits. The extra force being exerted by the heart to maintain blood flow can cause damage at junctures where larger arteries branch into smaller ones.

At these branches of the arterial system, it's as if a great river flows into many smaller streams. When a person's blood pressure is normal, the number of smaller streams is adequate to disperse the force of the larger stream.

With high blood pressure, that river moves with too much force into that series of small streams, creating what's called "shear force." The smaller streams become rapids and all the rushing blood cells scrape and wear away the lining of the artery.

Over time, these smaller arteries can be worn away to such an extent that the arterial wall itself can rupture, releasing blood directly, even into brain tissue. This results in a common form of stroke. Death is often the outcome.

The major coronary arteries are highly elastic and can suffer many insults to their structural integrity without impairing function. The same can't be said of the arterioles and their terminal ends, the capillaries. This is where most of the energy that keeps the body alive is exchanged; it's where the cells are fed and waste is eliminated.

Hypertension is a particular menace to the body's systems that are most dependent on the tiniest of arteries, also called arterioles or, in the case of the smallest of these, arterial capillaries. The brain, eyes, and kidneys are three such systems. Every neuron in the brain is intertwined with arterioles. The cones of the retinas are fed by millions of them. The tubules in the kidney's nephrons, as I mentioned before, are wrapped in climbing vines of them.

Capillaries are so small that just one red blood cell can pass through them at a time. They are far smaller than the thinnest of threads. As a result, it doesn't take much for a capillary's elasticity to wear out, become clogged by excess fat, or constrict to the point of uselessness. For this reason, declining mental function and kidney disease are often the consequence of prolonged, untreated or under-treated hypertension.

Fighting the Blood Pressure Battle

Knowing why you should fight the battle against hypertension is the first, all-important step. You may not be able to do anything about the genetic inheritance that predisposes you to essential hypertension, but you can do a great deal to mitigate its consequences.

Much of the hypertension epidemic we are living through today is due to excess salt in our diets. Going on a low-salt or no-salt diet is a major front in the battle against hypertension. Salt causes the body to retain fluid. The more fluid in the blood stream, the harder the heart has to work.

It's not easy to eliminate much of our salt intake from the diet, especially if we eat pre-packaged foods. A recent article that appeared on the front page of *The New York Times* showed how many packaged foods are little more than "salt-delivery devices."

Cheez-It crackers fall apart when much of the salt is removed and acquire a "medicinal" taste, the newspaper reports. As a Frito-Lay executive wrote in a 1979 internal memo: "Once a preference (for salt) is acquired most people do not change it, but simply obey it."

Here, then, are eight steps to slashing your blood-pressure risk:

- **Put down the salt shaker and learn to season your food with herbs and spices.** Try curry, fennel, and garlic, for instance. Eat fresh food — real food — as often as possible, not prepackaged food that can sit on a shelf for months or even years and still be "edible." Salt intake can be balanced, in part, by making sure you have enough magnesium, potassium, and calcium in your diet. These reduce the ill effects of salt. Magnesium widens blood vessels and is used on pregnant women who have high blood pressure. The dosages of these substances, however, are hard to calibrate. Magnesium can be taken until it causes diarrhea, then lower the dose. Calcium and magnesium are best when taken together. Be careful, though, because too much potassium — that is, excessive amounts — can be lethal to your kidneys. All of these substances should be taken in consultation with your doctor.

- **If you want to avoid taking drugs for hypertension or stop taking them, the most significant thing you can do is get down to your ideal body weight.** A loss of 10 pounds usually equates to the normal dosage of one medication. Many who suffer from hypertension see this condition completely vanish when they reach their ideal body weight — what you weighed, or close to it, in high school or college. Once again, exercise is crucial. Your cardiovascular system is alive and constantly changing. Exercise builds up the heart in the right way and helps restore elasticity to the arteries. The sequence of putting the cardiovascular system under exercise stress and then taking that stress away brings down blood pressure to what it would be if the person merely rested.

- **Stay away from stimulants like coffee, tea, sodas, alcohol, and cigarettes.** You simply cannot smoke. Your doctor can advise you as to whether your hypertension warrants cutting out all stimulants, or if you can still enjoy a cup of coffee in the morning. Many people sip diet sodas throughout the day. These have caffeine and can raise blood pressure significantly.

- **Make sure you are getting enough sleep, at least eight to 10 hours daily.** Sleep deprivation is a leading cause of hypertension because it puts the body under stress. If your loved ones complain about snoring or especially snorting and snuffling during the night, you may be suffering from sleep apnea — a rapid cycle of waking up many times at night, periods during which the heart may stop. Sleep apnea puts the body under tremendous stress and causes secondary hypertension.

- **Live below your means** so that you are not constantly stressed out about finances.

- **Don't forget to have fun!** Enjoying social times, particularly with people you know well, helps you cope with stress. Keeping a quiet time each day is also very important, whether that means time alone or, much better, in prayer.

- **Finally, if you are found to have hypertension and your physician prescribes medication, take it!** The information above should give you every reason to do so. Take your medication at least until you can change your diet and exercise patterns to achieve an ideal body weight. That will obviate the need, in many cases, for continuing such medication.

Many people feel energetic when their blood pressure is high and listless or fatigued when it returns to normal. I try to prescribe medication so that the person's blood pressure returns to normal not all at once but over a short span of time. This allows the person to adjust to what a normal blood pressure feels like.

Most people whose hypertension is treated adequately and with a gentle hand feel much better as a result. Employ every weapon available to win the blood pressure battle!

CHAPTER 13

The Bypass Option?
Always Get a Second Opinion

Imagine this scenario: In a game of doubles tennis, you were reaching for a backhand passing shot when all at once you were "doubled" over by chest pains. One look at you and your tennis partner ran for his cell phone to call 911. After what seemed like an eternity — but only lasted 12 minutes — you were on the way to the emergency room facing a far tougher opponent than the hackers across the net.

One doctor comes in, then another; the nurses are all over the place and people in scrubs called "techs" are monitoring an array of machines that apparently report that you are still alive, though no one in his right mind would call this living.

Eventually, a man enters wearing a surgical cap. He tells you that you need a triple bypass operation, and that it would be best to schedule one as soon as your condition allows. He'd be happy to be your surgeon, as he's worked on thousands of similar cases.

Given the surroundings, you are prepared to believe him. Except that, as the doctor walks out the door, one of the techs makes sure he's out of sight and then smirks. A nurse raises her brows and nods.

"What?" you say.

The tech's face turns to stone, but the nurse comes over and says, "It's always good to get a second opinion. I'd do that if I were you."

Are you being hustled? And if so, in what direction: toward bypass surgery or toward a different option? Aren't these people supposed to be straight with you? Don't they know your life is on the line?

This confusing situation confronts thousands of people each year, as more studies suggest that bypass surgery might not always be the best course of treatment. But how do you decide between having a bypass operation or less traumatic measures such as medication and lifestyle changes? And what are your options?

The bottom line is that bypass surgery should be considered a treatment of last resort. There are cases in which bypass surgery remains the best course. But those cases occur far less frequently today because of medical advances.

I recommend beginning with the least-traumatic, least-invasive measures possible. This is not merely a matter of kindness; less trauma is always better for a patient's long-term health.

If at all possible, you should involve loved ones and your primary care physician in the decision because those are the people who know you best and care about you most. If your condition is stable enough to allow it, take the time to get a second opinion. If you are already in the hospital, your insurance company probably will cover the extra cost. If you have been treated strictly on an outpatient basis, insurance might cover the extra cost, but you'll need to check.

Bypass surgery may be indicated for three groups:

1. **Critical heart disease.** Blockages of 75 percent or greater in at least three vessels, along with associated depressed left ventricular function. This refers to the heart's "ejection fraction," or its ability to discharge the blood in its chambers. If this ratio has fallen to less than 35 percent, you are a candidate for bypass surgery. Keep in mind that critical blockage must be present in three vessels. It's often the case that one vessel is almost totally blocked while the remaining vessels have less serious blockages. This allows for a different course of treatment.

2. **Critical left main artery disease of more than 75 percent.** These patients may be treated with bypass surgery, but don't necessarily need a bypass. These cases are challenging to diagnose, and treatment often depends on the skill of the physicians involved.

3. **Diabetics with three-vessel coronary artery disease.** The percentage of blockage in all three of a diabetic's vessels does not have to rise to the threshold of non-diabetics (i.e., 75 percent), because diabetics are less able to take advantage of less-invasive measures and lifestyle change.

Bypass surgery used to be regarded almost as a panacea, with patients undergoing multiple bypass surgeries over the course of their lives. But 20 years ago doctors had fewer options, and merely offered whatever help they could to patients with critical heart disease.

Today, we have other options. And if we do perform a bypass, we want the first surgery to be the last. The good news is that we've learned so much more about heart disease that, with the patient's cooperation, that outcome is possible.

Why Is Bypass the Last Resort?

There's no minimizing the trauma of a bypass surgery. Opening a patient's chest cavity like the door of a birdcage inevitably puts a tremendous stress on the whole body. The grafts (sections of good vessel substituted for blocked vessel) are usually taken from veins in the legs.

But those vessels were meant to support a lower carrying capacity — to be part of a lower blood pressure system — than the vessels near the heart. When they are grafted to the main arteries near the heart, they become part of a high pressure system. Also, the way the veins are dissected from the leg and then stretched to make them fit the graft can damage the tissue of the vessel.

Another bypass method is to redirect the right and left internal mammary arteries that feed the tissues over the breastplate. In this case, one or both arteries are separated painstakingly from the surrounding tissues and redirected to the heart.

The great plus of using the mammary arteries is that they are meant to be part of a high pressure system, so they don't inevitably close up. They also have enough sub-arteries branching off of them to continue feeding the tissues over the breastplate — at least in non-diabetic patients. Diabetics can only use one of their mammary arteries for a bypass; otherwise, the tissues over the breastplate don't receive adequate blood flow.

Even so, in triple, quadruple, or quintuple bypass procedures, human veins or pig vessels have to be used for the other grafts. Using internal mammary arteries is a much more difficult procedure — beyond the skill level of some surgeons. It's a time-consuming operation, and any increase in the duration of a surgery increases the risk. Any patient who opts to have the internal mammary arteries used for grafts must consider this.

All told, 15 percent of bypass surgeries fail within the first three months. Within 10 years, 50 percent of bypass grafts have plugged up.

Chances are that a bypass surgery will fail at some point. The surgery itself also carries the risk of sternal infections, stroke, and blood clots in the lungs.

And there are particular risks for patients 70 years or older. In order to perform bypass surgery, the surgeon assigns blood flow and respiration to a heart-lung machine. This allows the surgeon to work on a quiet heart that's no longer beating, and one that, drained of blood, goes from its normal globular shape to being flat as a pancake. This "quiet field" is the ideal landscape for the delicate incisions and suturing that must be done on grafts.

Unfortunately, heart-lung machines carry the risk of what's commonly known as "pump brain." No one knows exactly why, but patients who are put on heart-lung machines can suffer neurological damage, such as confusion or loss of memory — and in the elderly, there is a possibility of introducing or exacerbating dementia. An elderly patient could undergo a bypass operation that seems a resounding success, ridding him of heart disease completely — only to quickly decline into a dementia that results in death.

In addition, during bypass surgery the lungs are deflated and tubes are inserted into the bottom of each lung to drain fluid. After surgery, the lungs remain partially collapsed. For this reason, bypass patients are urged before surgery to take deep breaths as soon as they wake up from the anesthesia — their lungs need clearing.

As someone who supervised the heart transplant program at the Medical College of Virginia, I have the utmost respect for the tremendous skills of heart surgeons. These men and women perform life-saving procedures that demand gifts few people possess. However, there are other options.

The Move Toward Interventional Medicine

Unfortunately, interventional cardiologists (my specialty) are not all created equal. Some are far more adept at handling complicated cases. The less skilled a patient's interventional cardiologist, the better the odds the patient will end up in the hands of a surgeon.

And in my experience, many patients who have suffered a cardiac event do not need the last-ditch intervention of a surgeon. They can now be treated through balloon angioplasty and the insertion of stents.

For example, a patient may have three-vessel heart disease but only one of the blockages is the source of immediate problems. A gifted interventional cardiologist will recommend addressing the major blockage with balloon angioplasty and the insertion of a stent — procedures that will see the patient home in a couple of days, feeling much better. A less-proficient doctor might worry that his skills are inadequate to carry out such a procedure.

The talented interventionalist is also more likely to take a "wait and see approach" as to whether (once the major blockage has been addressed) the minor blockages can be remedied through medication and lifestyle adjustment.

It's also a matter of keeping up with the latest medical research and advancements. For instance, when balloon angioplasty was introduced in 1977, it was much less reliable and effective than it is today.

Back then, doctors inflated the balloon within the artery, breaking up the plaque blocking it, and hoped the artery would "remodel," or assume a shape and form that was more favorable. Often, these arteries did just that, as the body seemed to recognize the chance to heal itself. But not always.

Sometimes, the arteries would seem fine in the catheterization lab, then close as soon as the patient reached the recovery room. We soon learned that there is a "rebound effect": Like other elastic materials, arteries that have been opened with balloon angioplasty contract after having been expanded.

Balloon angioplasty still helped because only a slight improvement in the artery produced increased blood flow. However, it could break up the plaque in a way that produced thrombosis — clotting of the blood — which could lead to heart attack or stroke. Arteries treated with balloon angioplasty alone re-block (a process called restenosis) at a rate of 30 to 50 percent.

Nowadays, the procedure is complemented with the insertion of stents, hollow tubes made of wire mesh that keep the artery open after the balloon has been removed. With the advent of stents, doctors can remodel the artery after the angioplasty, ensuring free blood flow.

There are still problems with stents, however. They can cause irritation to the arterial wall, and the body's immune system responds to this irritation prompting the natural lining of the artery — the endothelium — to absorb the stent; within six months, the artery manages to line the stent with its own cells.

Usually, the immune process stops at this point, and the stent has a lining of living cells, allowing the vessel to function perfectly. In some cases, though, the body's immune system keeps going, and the arterial wall grows around and eventually into the stent until it becomes blocked.

The first type of stent, the uncoated stent, becomes blocked again 15 to 30 percent of the time. The way in which restenosis occurs can be likened to the formation of scar tissue. Usually, if you cut your skin, a virtually imperceptible scar will trace out the healed wound. In some cases, however, a scar will form. Here, the scar tissue proliferates, turns pink, and exaggerates the size of the old injury.

The irritation to the arterial wall caused by an uncoated stent also may cause a blood clot, which can precipitate heart attack or stroke. For this reason, people with stents must take an antiplatelet medication such as clopidogrel (Plavix) for six months, as well as daily aspirin.

We now have a second type of stent, coated stents, designed to suppress cell growth around and inside the stent. These are also called "drug-eluting stents" because they "elute" or give off a drug that suppresses the body's immune response, which prevents the stent from being overgrown and forming blockages in the artery.

Coated stents remain open indefinitely, but because they suppress the body's immune response they are even more prone than non-coated stents to promote blood clots. This risk rises substantially in the event of surgery for another condition. For example, if a patient with a coated stent needs to have his gall bladder removed, the chances of gall bladder surgery producing a blood clot are substantially higher.

Personally, I prefer the use of uncoated stents. If I can monitor a patient closely, and the patient takes prescribed medications and actively pursues lifestyle modification, including proper diet and exercise, then there is a great chance for success without the need for extended drug therapy. Restenosis usually occurs within the first three to six months for non-coated stents.

Monthly appointments and the administration of a stress test six months after insertion can help gauge whether there's been an adverse reaction to the non-coated stent.

My preference for uncoated vs. coated, however, has exceptions. Diabetics are far more prone to reclosure of a stent, and for that reason they should be treated with coated stents.

Lifestyle Change Can Beat Heart Disease

The best-case scenario is where neither bypass surgery nor balloon angioplasty and stenting need be used. Many non-acute cases of heart disease can be treated with medications and lifestyle changes alone.

Non-acute cases are those where the patient has not suffered a major cardiac event, but does suffer from conditions such as stable angina (chest pains brought on by activity or stress), blockages that have been detected through a positive stress test, and even minor heart attacks.

The 2007 COURAGE study, conducted by the American College of Cardiology Scientific Sessions, compared the cases of more than 2,000 patients with one-vessel disease, stable angina, and a positive stress test (meaning a test that indicated the presence of heart disease). Half of the recipients received balloon angioplasty and stents, and half were treated only with medications and lifestyle modification (diet, exercise, and stress reduction techniques). The incidence of heart attack was the same in both groups, though those with stents received greater relief from angina.

What we are learning is that medication and lifestyle change can accomplish more in the reversal of heart disease than once was thought possible. Someone who is truly committed to eating a plant-based diet, walking an hour a day, investing more time in family, and modifying their work schedule can see significant rejuvenation of their arterial system.

The blockages won't disappear, but they can be improved modestly with the right medications and lifestyle changes, allowing blood flow to improve dramatically. Functionally, heart disease can become a thing of the past.

As you assess your situation and the treatments recommended, keep in mind how you live your life. If you are retired, live close to your doctor or a hospital, and have a predictable routine, then you are in a position to take a conservative approach.

If, however, you are still in mid-career, and don't know whether you'll be in the Grand Canyon or Timbuktu next week, then you and your doctors should be more aggressive. After all, you don't want to find yourself in the Outback with chest pains.

To deal with heart disease and all other serious conditions, cultivate a relationship with your primary care physician. Every time a doctor sees a patient, he comes to know the whole person better. The doctor knows how the patient reacts to stress, what type of support network the patient has, and the types of care to which the patient responds most positively.

The whole psycho-social dynamic of the doctor-patient relationship is crucial when it comes to making big medical decisions — like how to address heart disease.

CHAPTER 14

Unclog Your Arteries
Without Surgery

Interventional medicine is a branch of cardiology that uses nonsurgical procedures to treat heart disease — specifically atherosclerosis, a condition in which the walls of an artery become lined with fat, cholesterol, and other substances. Eventually, the artery becomes so coated that blood cannot flow, and the blood vessel needs to be opened. A stenting procedure is a noninvasive (nonsurgical) method interventional physicians use to open the artery.

It's rare for me to ever send a patient for bypass. In the past, before stenting became an option, I used to send three people a week for bypass surgery. Today, that number has decreased to about three people per year. I was fortunate to begin my training when stents were coming into mainstream use. I've always been aware of the benefits nonsurgical interventions offer to the patient, and it has been ingrained in the way I treat my patients.

The history of treating heart disease with interventional medicine goes back to the 1970s, and starts with Dr. Andreas Gruentzig. Prior to his work with interventional techniques, Dr. Gruentzig had been experimenting with balloon catheters in Germany, but he encountered skepticism from his colleagues regarding his proposed procedure.

In 1969, he moved his research to Switzerland, and developed balloon catheters that were small enough to fit inside coronary arteries, as well as being strong enough to crush arterial plaque against the artery walls, thus clearing the way for blood to flow. In 1975, he presented his research at an American Heart Association meeting, where, just as in Germany, he was met with skepticism. However, a few physicians were intrigued by the idea.

In 1977, Dr. Gruentzig, along with the American physician Richard Myers, performed the first ever coronary angioplasty — often called balloon angioplasty — in San Francisco. The patient had been prepped for bypass, and his chest was open when the physicians completed the procedure.

After the procedure, Dr. Gruentzig returned to Zurich and created a catheter that could be snaked through a patient's coronary arteries, and the first truly noninvasive (nonsurgical) procedure — percutaneous transluminal coronary angioplasty (PTCA) — was complete.

Although he performed the intervention successfully, physicians in Zurich did not accept his methods, and were not helpful in efforts to find suitable patients for this intervention. Dr. Gruentzig began searching for a more supportive environment in the United States.

Fortunately, a number of cardiologists from Emory University School of Medicine in Atlanta, Ga., had attended a course he taught in Europe. When they learned of his desire to practice in the United States, they were able to secure a faculty spot at Emory.

Dr. Gruentzig was named director of interventional cardiovascular medicine at Emory, where he continued to work until his death in 1985.

But the use of PTCA was just beginning. And because I was doing my medical training and research during this time, I have a different perspective on these procedures than the doctors who are being trained today.

I saw how nonsurgical procedures worked when opening blocked arteries (called an angioplasty), why they worked, the difficulties with the procedure, and why it was such a leap forward compared to surgery. Those of us who trained during that time looked at anatomy differently, handled cases differently, and gained a lot of experience in solving the problems that the procedure could cause.

We would begin by threading a balloon through an artery in either an arm or leg, and then inflate it at the site of blockage. Although the balloon was quite capable of opening, or dilating, the artery, once the balloon was removed, the artery would recoil like a rubber band and cause the walls to close.

This was a huge issue, as the goal of the procedure was to break up the plaque in the hope that the artery would return to its original, open shape. Sometimes even after the procedure, the arteries would close up, restricting blood flow. Another issue we ran into was that during the procedure the artery could fracture and develop a blood clot, or a calcification from the plaque could break off.

One technique we tried was called a "perfusion balloon." In this procedure, we used a type of balloon that had holes which allowed continuous blood flow while doctors worked to dilate the artery.

Perfusion balloon insertion typically took three to six hours to perform, and during that time doctors gained a lot of experience in how PTCA affects damaged arteries, as well as the difficulties in reaching a successful outcome for the patient.

In those early days, while we were performing PTCAs, the operating room was always ready for cases in which the artery closed down and the patient needed immediate bypass surgery — because at that time there was no other interventional option.

Then stents appeared, and radically changed the treatment of blocked arteries.

What Is a Stent?

A stent is essentially a mesh cage that is placed inside the artery wall to help it hold its shape. If magnified, it would look like chicken wire rolled into a small tube. The first use of a stent occurred in 1987, although the FDA didn't approve the device for widespread use until 1994.

As I noted earlier, there are two types of stents: noncoated, which is more commonly used; and the coated, or drug-eluting stent, which emits an immunosuppressant drug to inhibit cell growth (this helps in keeping the artery clear for blood to flow through).

During the procedure, the patient is awake, but sedated. (It is generally an overnight procedure, and most patients go home the next day.) The stent surrounds the angioplasty balloon and is threaded into place in the artery through a small catheter in an artery in the leg. The physician uses contrast dye and X-ray images to guide the balloon and stent into place.

When the balloon and stent have reached the area of blockage, the balloon is inflated, and the stent that surrounds it is pressed into the artery wall. The balloon is then deflated and removed, leaving the stent in place to hold the artery open like a scaffold.

There are a number of concerns when inserting a noncoated stent into a diseased artery. First of all, the metal in the stents can cause blood to coagulate, triggering a risk of blood clots. For this reason, all patients who have stents inserted are prescribed clopidogrel (Plavix) or prasugrel (Effient) — antiplatelet drugs that inhibit the formation of blood clots — along with daily aspirin.

Another issue that can arise has to do with the body's natural defense mechanisms. Ironically, the body's immune system can be too effective. During a normal immune response, a stent is viewed as a foreign object, and the cells that line the inside of the artery (called the endothelium) try to absorb the stent — an action that is similar to what happens when you get a splinter.

For most people, the tissue grows only to a certain point and then stops. However, in some, the immune reaction kicks into high gear and grows so much scar tissue that it ultimately blocks the artery itself.

It takes three to six months before thickening of this scar tissue is apparent. If the scar tissue becomes too thick, a patient will need to have the artery reopened; another stent will be placed within the first stent. Radiation may be necessary to remove scar tissue.

To resolve this issue, another type of stent became available in 2004: the coated or drug-eluting stent. These stents are coated with a drug that suppresses the body's immune system function so that scar tissue won't grow and block the artery.

The drug is effective in up to 98 percent of cases. However, because the rate of tissue growth is slowed, these stents are more prone to cause blood clots (stent thrombosis). In the past, patients who received them had to remain on antiplatelet drugs for at least a year.

There is some debate about using coated stents versus noncoated stents.

Diabetics, women, and smokers are considered good candidates for coated stents because their vessels are smaller and may have a quicker recurrence of blockage, and there may be concerns with clotting.

A noncoated stent might be used on someone who only has one problem area and has larger arteries. It's up to the doctor to determine what is appropriate for each particular patient. I haven't seen any strong evidence to support the automatic use of either stent in particular populations.

There are still patients today who receive balloon angioplasty. If the patient is a candidate, and the procedure seems to hold, doctors will leave it at that. We examine all the blockages and decide whether the blockage needs angioplasty, a stent or, rarely, a bypass.

Sometimes a patient will receive a combination of procedures, as some of their atherosclerosis sites may be more critical than others (we call these "culprit sites"). I try to always use the interventional procedures first, recommending diet and lifestyle modifications, as well as medications, to prevent the need for invasive — or even non-invasive — procedures.

Patients who need these procedures should make sure that their doctor has a thorough knowledge of interventional medicine and a long track record of successful procedures.

There is no denying that stents have improved treatment for athero-sclerosis. For example, arteries treated with a balloon angioplasty alone will experience additional blockage in 30 percent of cases. The use of stents has reduced the recurrence of blockage to 15 percent of cases.

Regaining Your Health

The interventional procedure is only the beginning of treatment. The procedure solves the immediate health risk, but it does not resolve the ongoing issues that caused the problem in the first place.

Patients must maintain a healthy lifestyle through a controlled diet and exercise program. This is how you regain control of your health.

The good news is that this goal is 100 percent possible to achieve. Heart disease is not a death sentence; patients are not doomed to have a heart attack simply because they have had a stent put in.

I like to see patients on a monthly basis for a full year after an intervention. This is crucial to ensure that we are addressing the issues that caused the need for the intervention in the first place.

During the first six months, every patient receives cholesterol and anti-platelet medications, and they are encouraged to stick to a low-fat, low-cholesterol, vegetarian diet. The first months are critical to ensuring that the artery heals properly around the stent.

After six months, I add meat, in moderation, back into patients' diets, and help them taper off their medications once they reach the target therapeutic levels for hypertension, cholesterol and weight.

As doctors, we are trained to focus on family history, lifestyle, and the presence of diseases such as diabetes. But we sometimes under-play the role of stress in our patients' — and our own — health.

Heart attacks affect police officers, firefighters, CEOs, and physicians more than any other working populations. Continuous stress can increase blood pressure and release hormones that can affect clotting and increase the amount of cholesterol in the blood, causing plaque buildup.

The lesson is that we need to be more reasonable about the pressures we put on ourselves. While the body has mechanisms in place for "fight or flight" survival stress, it was not built for continuous stress.

We are now seeing a trend of early onset heart disease, and doctors are performing more interventional procedures on people in their 30s than ever before. This is mostly due to dietary choices, smoking, and history of drug use. The youngest patient I've treated was only 28. Why? Because he chose to eat fast food every day, multiple times a day.

Your health is a responsibility. It's a responsibility to your family, your children, and to anyone who depends on you. And keep in mind that there is a lifetime of recovery that goes hand-in-hand with a non-invasive procedure that involves complete lifestyle modifications, all of which you can implement in your life today.

CHAPTER 15

You're Having a Heart Attack — What Should You Do?

A s with many other forms of medical knowledge, if you are get-ting information about what a heart attack is like from TV or the movies, you could be in big trouble.

Doctors call it the "Hollywood Heart Attack." This is when an actor grabs his chest, drops to his knees and leaves no doubt about what is happening. Actor Redd Foxx was famous for his "fake" heart attacks on the 1970s sitcom *Sanford and Son*.

Ironically, Foxx did die of a heart attack on the set of a different TV series. Everyone thought he was acting, but he was having a real heart attack. There's no way to know if Foxx could have survived, but there's no doubt that precious time was lost in getting him to the hospital.

How do you know if you or someone you are with is having a heart attack? What should you do in either case?

The truth is this: It can be hard to tell what is happening in case of a heart attack; not all heart attack symptoms are alike.

People often react to heart attack symptoms with denial; the time that is lost before getting help can be the difference between life and death. In addition, people often make the wrong decisions even if they understand they are having a heart attack; getting the right kind of help, within the right time frame, will determine how a person spends the rest of their life.

The good news is that heart emergencies can be treated. A heart attack can be stopped in its tracks and you can go on to lead a normal life — but only if you know what to do and follow through quickly.

A heart attack, also called a myocardial infarction (MI), happens when blood flow to the heart is blocked. It is usually triggered by the rupture of plaque buildup inside a coronary artery, which causes a clot. When the artery is blocked, the area of the heart it supplies is deprived of blood and oxygen. That part of the heart begins to die.

When heart muscle dies, the damage is permanent. Early treatment can reduce or reverse the amount of damage the heart muscle suffers. Minutes count! And I mean that literally.

For anyone having a heart attack, immediate medical attention is critical for two reasons: Most of the damage done by a heart attack occurs during the first few hours; treatment given during that time can help mitigate permanent heart muscle damage.

Cardiac arrest, a sudden loss of heart function due to an abnormal heartbeat, is a danger during the first few hours of a heart attack. Without a defibrillator to shock the heart, death occurs in minutes.

Despite what many people think, heart attack and cardiac arrest are not the same thing. A heart attack refers to the death of heart muscle tissue due to loss of blood supply. Cardiac arrest, which can be brought on by a heart attack, is the total loss of heart function due to electrical malfunction of the heart.

When the heart stops, blood doesn't flow to the brain or the rest of the body. A person will collapse, lose consciousness, and stop breathing. The American Heart Association reports that every year about 500,000 Americans die from cardiac arrest before they can get to the hospital.

The Symptoms of a Heart Attack

Unlike the dramatic Hollywood Heart Attack, many heart attacks start slowly. Often, a person doesn't even realize what is happening. Symptoms also vary, so even someone who has already had a heart attack may experience different symptoms.

Here are the things that can indicate a heart attack:
- Pain, pressure, or constriction in the chest
- Discomfort that spreads to the shoulders, arm, back, neck, or jaw
- Nausea or vomiting
- Indigestion, heartburn, or a choking feeling
- Shortness of breath
- Sweating
- Rapid or irregular heartbeats
- Vague feeling of illness
- Anxiety or a feeling of doom
- Dizziness, weakness, or lightheadedness
- Sudden, overwhelming fatigue

As you can see, that's a lot of symptoms. Many are indistinct, and could easily indicate another condition, such as indigestion, muscle strain, the onset of flu, or an adverse reaction to medication.

However, if you are over 50 and have risk factors for heart disease — such as being a smoker, diabetic, overweight or have high cholesterol, high blood pressure, or a family history of heart problems — you must take the symptoms seriously.

Of course, you can have a heart attack even if you don't have risk factors and are not over 50. In my own case, I had a blocked artery at age 48. When the pain started in my shoulder, I thought I had strained a muscle. The pain was uncomfortable but not severe, so I did nothing about it.

But the next day it was much worse. Still, it took me 24 hours to put together what was happening and get treatment. In hindsight, I should have gotten checked out the first day.

If you have any of the risk factors for heart disease and develop any combination of those symptoms, you have to call 911 immediately. Even if you don't have the risk factors, spending hours wondering if the discomfort will go away is a waste of precious time — and denial of what is happening can kill you.

Remember, the clock starts ticking when the symptoms start, not when they become unbearable. The first hour is often referred to as the "Golden Hour" because there is still time to revive the oxygen-starved heart. The sooner blood flow is restored, the less damage is done.

Do not drive yourself or have someone else drive you to the hospital. Call 911. Cardiac arrest is a possibility when you are having a heart attack. If that happens, you will need an electronic defribrillator to restart the heart. Paramedics will have a defibrillator on hand. That way you can receive lifesaving treatment at home or on the way to the hospital, if necessary.

While you are waiting for the ambulance to come, chew two regular tablets of aspirin. This will start working to thin the blood clot or slow the buildup. Do not take aspirin if you are allergic to it.

If you are on any medication, set it out for emergency personnel to see. If you take nitroglycerin, take it as directed. Do not take someone else's nitroglycerin.

I always advise people that if you think someone you are with is having a heart attack, don't discuss it. The person will most likely deny their symptoms and may even be embarrassed. The best thing to do is excuse yourself and call 911. Getting paramedics on the way as soon as possible can save a life.

If the person passes out, you will need to perform CPR until help arrives. Call 911 and put them on speakerphone so they can talk you through the chest compressions. If the person wakes up, they may be confused and alarmed. Do your best to keep them calm and warm. Then let them know that help is on the way. Have them turn onto their side so that their breathing won't be obstructed if they vomit.

If you are in a public place, find out if a defibrillator is available. Many airports, train stations, universities, restaurants, casinos, and sports facilities have portable defibrillators on-site and staff that is trained to use them. They are called "automated external defibrillators" or AEDs. These are not the same units that hospitals and paramedics use, but they can save a life in an emergency.

AEDs are very user-friendly. They have an electronic voice prompter that talks users through each step, even giving instructions on how to connect the electrodes to the patient. The device is programmed to diagnose a person's heart rhythm and determine if a shock is needed.

Automatic models will administer the shock; semi-automatic models tell the user to push a button for the shock. Many lives have been saved with these devices.

What Happens at the Hospital

Once paramedics arrive, they will assess the condition of the patient. They may call the emergency department to consult with a physician before stabilizing the patient and preparing him or her for transport to a hospital.

In larger cities, the paramedics may be able to do an electrocardiogram (EKG) on the scene or during transport. This test measures the electrical activity of the heart. If a heart attack is indicated, the paramedics will take the patient to the nearest heart center and call ahead to the emergency room so that the hospital is ready as soon as the patient arrives.

If an EKG has not been done before the patient reaches the hospital, it will be done immediately. Aspirin will be given if it has not already. The patient will also get oxygen, if needed, and an IV line so that fluids and medication can be administered. Pain medication will be given as necessary.

The EKG will determine if the patient has a partially or completely blocked artery. A complete blockage means the patient will need cardiac catheterization (insertion of a tube) to have the blockage opened with a balloon angioplasty.

The time it takes to get the angioplasty done in an emergency setting is called "door to balloon" time. It starts as soon as the patient gets to the hospital. The national benchmark is 90 minutes or less, so heart centers will be on alert to initiate the procedure as soon as they determine it is needed.

The same goes for giving clot-busting drugs when there is a partial blockage in the artery. This is called the "door to drug" time; the sooner the medication is given, the better. If paramedics can transmit an EKG to the hospital and the drug is indicated, it might even be given in the ambulance.

Once emergency procedures have been completed, the patient will be transferred to the Coronary Care Unit (CCU), where he or she can be monitored and evaluated. This unit focuses on relieving pain and reducing strain on the heart.

The patient will start out on strict bed rest and a restricted diet, but will be eased back onto regular food and normal activity. Depending on the severity of the heart attack, the patient will go home anywhere from a few days to a week.

Life After a Heart Attack

A cardiologist will provide thorough at-home instructions for recovering from a heart attack. There will be medications, dietary restrictions, and follow up appointments. The patient will likely be enrolled in a program to gradually increase exercise and normal activities.

But the fact remains that a heart attack is a life-changing event. Surviving it is not the end of the experience — it's just the beginning. Most people will make a physical recovery, but many will be surprised by the emotional effects of a heart attack.

It is natural to be shocked by what has happened. Common feelings include:

- **Fear.** Often, people who have suffered a heart attack are afraid that it will happen again. They worry about going back to work, wonder if they will ever feel in control again, and feel anxiety about the pain coming back. They may think that any exercise could be fatal. These are all normal fears that people have to work through.

- **Depression.** This feeling is so common that it is actually considered part of the recovery process. The fear and anxiety over having the heart attack take a while to come to terms with. People may feel like their life is over. It's not.

- **Anger.** If you have led a healthy lifestyle, you may even feel angry. After all, how could a person do "all the right things" and still have a heart attack? It doesn't seem fair, but anger is stressful and needs to be dealt with.

- **Guilt.** If you did have some bad habits like smoking and not exercising, you may think the heart attack was your fault. But guilt doesn't make anything better. Focus on making the changes you need to.

The important thing is to recognize that recovery from a heart attack will be *both* physical and emotional. It's impossible to ignore the emotional roller coaster. Take advantage of the support of your family and friends. Take things one day at a time.

If depression becomes overwhelming, get help. Your doctor can adjust your medications and recommend counseling. Many people have gone through the same thing and support groups are available where you can hear how others have dealt with adjusting to life after a heart attack. You really are not alone.

The key to surviving a heart attack is quick treatment. The most important thing you can do is to know the symptoms. And when you feel or see those symptoms, *do not delay!* Call 911 immediately.

Statistics show that most people wait and wonder about the symptoms for a good 2 1/2 hours before going to the hospital.

You may be unsure because it doesn't seem like the typical Hollywood Heart Attack. But it is possible to prevent much of the damage of a heart attack and go on to lead a normal life. When it comes to a heart attack, time is life.

PART THREE

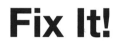

Fix It!

CHAPTER 16

Dr. Crandall's 3-Point Plan for Heart Health

Every day, I see people whose faces are creased with worry — they are people who have had a heart attack and fear that another one could kill them. But they start to relax when I give them the good news that they can, in fact, prevent that next heart attack. And they can hardly believe it when I tell them that if they follow my recommendations, they can actually reverse the heart disease and feel better than they have in years.

"What's the secret?" they wonder, sometimes out loud.

Well, here it is, in two words: "Get moving!" That's right, physical activity really is the "fountain of youth," and the path to that fountain is right outside your door.

We all know that a sedentary lifestyle is not healthy, but you may not realize just how bad it is. The human body is built for action, so lounging on the couch or sitting in front of the computer all day can result in a set of conditions — fat collecting around the abdomen, high blood pressure, cholesterol levels that are out of whack, and even diabetes — that significantly raise your risk for coronary heart disease.

Consider a large-group study by epidemiologist Alpa V. Patel, published in the *Journal of Epidemiology* in 2010. Patel and his research team tracked 53,440 men and 69,776 women, all of whom were healthy when the study started. After 14 years, the people who were the most sedentary were most likely to have died — and the cause usually was heart disease.

But here's the good news: Another study, published in 2010 in *Circulation*, looked at a group of 5,314 men, ages 65 to 92, and found that being active and fit cut their death rate by 38 percent — and the fittest of the group reduced their risk of dying by 61 percent!

I can testify personally to the truth of these statistics from my experiences with my own patients. Those who stay the healthiest — even if they are in their 80s or 90s — are the walkers.

The best thing people can do for their hearts, regardless of age, is to follow a program of daily, moderate exercise.

As I have noted, I face my own battle with heart disease, and I know the difference that keeping fit makes in my own life.

But even if I didn't have research or my patients to turn to, all I would need to do is observe history to know the best method for preventing heart disease. You might recall that I'm an old anthropology student, so I know that although heart disease is our most common killer today, it used to be rare.

Consider prehistoric man: He spent his days walking in search of food. But society evolved over millennia, and heart disease became more common — but only for the upper class because they had the luxury of being sedentary.

Then the Industrial Revolution changed life for everyone. Machines took the place of manual labor, and we took to traveling in cars, trains, and planes. And it's even worse in the computer age. We no longer even have to walk to the mailbox; we just zip off an e-mail.

Every little reason that we've had for keeping active has vanished, and we are paying for it with our health.

Because we no longer engage in active lives out of necessity, we must find ways to build physical activity into our daily routines to keep our hearts in good working order. That's why I've created "Dr. Crandall's 3-Point Plan to Keep Your Heart Young." It contains everything you need to know to get yourself active and keep your heart healthy.

Here's the plan in a nutshell:

1. **Walk Heart Disease Away**
2. **Retain Muscle Mass**
3. **Activity Trumps Stress**

Step 1. Walk Heart Disease Away

I walk for a full hour every day. I know this sounds simple, but don't fool yourself: Walking for 60 minutes each day requires commitment. But the benefits you reap will change your life.

Walking is an aerobic exercise, which means your heartbeat is raised for a sustained period of time. You may have heard that 30 minutes, a few times per week, is sufficient to keep you healthy. I disagree.

In fact, the reason those experts limit their recommendations to 30 minutes a few times per week is because they don't think that people will have the discipline to walk for a full hour every day. I have more faith.

Still, an hour per day can seem like a daunting task. I usually tell my patients to start with 20 minutes each day for two weeks, then advance to 40 minutes each day for another two weeks. After a month of warming up, they are ready to make the commitment to walking a full hour every day.

I believe that once people understand the biology behind walking an hour every day, and appreciate how it can improve their overall health — indeed, their lives — they will make the commitment.

Don't Forget Your Second Wind — When you wake up in the morning, or whenever you start to walk, your body has a built-in reserve of energy that lasts for about 30 minutes. The key is to continue walking past that 30-minute mark and tap into the body's collateral circulatory system.

Do you remember when you were young, and as you kept running, you got that exhilarating "second wind" feeling? Well, that's not all in your head. It's actually your body adjusting once it has gone through its built-in energy reserve. And the results are remarkable.

We're all familiar with the body's circulatory system, which consists of the vessels and muscles that control the blood flow throughout the body. The components of this system include the heart, arteries, veins, and capillaries.

What you may not know is that your body also has what's called a "collateral circulatory system," a microscopic network of blood vessels that ordinarily remain closed. However, with sustained physical activity — such as a daily, hour-long walk — these vessels open and become enlarged, forming an alternate network to bring blood to your heart. When these vessels open, it causes the "second wind" feeling of prolonged, aerobic exercise.

In addition, this blood flow can detour around blockages and relieve angina (chest pain that comes from heart disease) or even help to prevent a heart attack.

But that's not all that one-hour walk does. As you continue beyond the 30-minute mark, your body pumps up its production of nitric oxide, a gas that is credited with many benefits, such as helping keep arteries clean of plaque, as well as widening the arteries and keeping them supple. Each of these actions helps lower blood pressure, decreasing the risk of both heart attack and stroke.

Study: Take 10,000 Steps — But wait, as TV pitchmen say, there's more! As you continue to walk, your body goes through many beneficial processes, such as breaking down the fat in your liver and revving up your metabolism, which converts the sugar in your blood into energy more efficiently.

Study after study shows that regular walking helps prevent diabetes (or manage your blood sugar better if you already have the disease). For instance, a study published in the January issue of the *British Medical Journal* found that people who walked 10,000 steps a day as a form of exercise had a sharply reduced risk for diabetes. And how long does it take to walk 10,000 steps a day? About one hour.

Research presented at the American College of Cardiology's annual meeting provided definitive evidence that staying fit keeps your heart young. It is well known that muscle mass diminishes with aging. But this study, which looked at people older than 65, found that the hearts of those who stayed the most active looked more youthful than even the hearts of people aged 24 to 35.

In addition, the heart muscles in these study subjects were flexible. That meant that these older exercisers were less likely to develop diastolic heart failure, a condition in which the heart is unable to pump efficiently enough to keep up with the demands of the body.

Walking Is Just the Beginning — Why do I recommend walking instead of other activities? Over the years, I've kept track of my patients; I've watched tennis players develop shoulder problems, and runners cope with bad knees and hips. But when you walk, you can get all the benefits of aerobic exercise without putting undue strain on your joints.

Want to add variety to your exercise plan? Swimming is great, of course, but even if you don't swim, don't overlook the water. Check with health clubs or local pools for water aerobics classes.

When I get home from work, I make sure to add an additional activity period to the day as well. So, after dinner, this means I hop on my stationary bike, or perhaps I take a swim, or even take another walk. The idea is to keep moving.

Before you start any physical activity program, consult your physician. Most people can manage a short walk and build up from there, unless they have serious health problems. But it's always best to be safe.

Step 2. Build Muscle Mass

Although sustained aerobic activity is the cornerstone of my plan — because it builds up your cardiovascular system, which leads to endurance, lower blood pressure, and better heart health — this is not the only type of exercise your body craves. For optimal health, you need to build muscle mass.

Once we pass age 50, our sex hormone levels drop (testosterone in men, estrogen in women), which causes muscle mass to diminish.

When this happens, muscle is replaced with fat, and the flabby result shows in the mirror.

Regular strength training (also called resistance training) builds muscle and decreases the losses that are normally experienced with aging. Muscle tissue is very active and has high-energy requirements. This means that the more muscle you have (compared to fat), the more calories you can consume without gaining weight.

And there also are practical advantages to having more muscle mass.

Added muscle tissue helps maintain strength and bolster endurance. Muscle allows you to do the things you love to do, such as bowling, gardening, or even playing with the grandkids.

That's why it is so important to build strength training into your daily schedule.

Keep It Interesting — When I first present my physical activity recommendations to my patients, they are generally very agreeable. As I said, they've often just had a heart attack and are scared, so they'll agree to anything.

But time passes, and their attitude changes. After all, we all lead busy lives, and finding the time to exercise on a daily basis is difficult.

But this is your *life* we are talking about. Start off the day with that walk, or write your time at the gym into your appointment book. Discipline yourself to build this type of activity into your day, every day. Remember, heart disease is progressive; it never stops. So you cannot stop, either. You need to stay active to beat it.

Here, then, are some ways to keep your activity program interesting:

- **Build in variety.** Find a local walking track or bike trail, drive to a park or a different neighborhood to explore a different environment — keep it interesting.

- **Vary your program according to the season.** You need to find a way to exercise year-round, whether you do so at home, at the gym, outdoors in good weather, or at a mall if it's rainy. (No pausing or window-shopping!)

- **Walk with your spouse or a friend.** But make sure that you're both committed to walking because chatting will slow you down. This is true, also, of walking with your dog. Save that type of walking for the additional activity because you won't reap all of the benefits of your hour-long walk.

- **Give ballroom dancing a whirl.** Some of my oldest, happiest, and healthiest patients are ballroom dancers; they relish both the activity and the sociability that comes along with it.

By the way, my wife is as committed to exercise as I am. Normally, we don't exercise together, though. My wife prefers running rather than walking, so she runs five miles, six days a week. Twice a day, she goes for a 20-minute walk with our dogs.

Step 3. Activity Trumps Stress

Researchers have long suspected that stress plays a role in heart disease, but they hadn't pinpointed exactly how stress was affecting the heart until recently. Now they know that stress can be caused by cigarettes, fatty foods, sugary treats, and the other confirmed causes of heart disease.

Here's how it works: Stress is the body's response to an imminent threat. Once again, we can think back to our prehistoric ancestors to understand just how this process works.

Imagine a prehistoric man out in the open, searching for food, when a saber-toothed tiger suddenly comes across his path. His body had to spring into action to avoid becoming food himself.

Automatically, his adrenal glands started emitting hormones, including adrenalin and cortisol, to quicken his heart and get blood pumping to his legs to enable him to escape. This is what's known as the "fight-or-flight" response.

Although we aren't likely to encounter any saber-toothed tigers as we go about our daily life nowadays, we do get into stressful situations, such as fights with our bosses or money troubles. In those cases, our adrenal glands keep churning out hormones. As a result, these hormones, particularly cortisol, remain in our bloodstream too long.

Beating 'Fight or Flight' — Now here's the connection. As you'll recall, the formation of plaque in the arteries is the hallmark of heart disease. This plaque not only causes blockages but also damages walls of blood vessels.

Unfortunately, the body's reaction is to send white blood cells to fight that plaque. The result is inflammation, which can cause a bit of the plaque to break off and head further down through the blood to the artery, where it can cause a blockage that results in a heart attack.

The body does have ways to dampen this inflammatory response. However — and this is where stress comes in — the cortisol released as a "fight-or-flight" response blocks the body's dampening mechanism, thereby fueling the inflammation as well.

Fortunately, you can blunt the "flight-or-fight" response by being active. When you exercise, your body produces endorphins, which are hormones that act as natural mood elevators. This is how activity alleviates depression. Over time, the natural suppression of cortisol also will cause a drop in blood pressure.

By sticking to this three-step plan, you can reap the benefits of activity, which not only can forestall heart disease but also will have you feeling healthier than you have in years.

CHAPTER 17

Reversing Heart Disease for Life

Yes, heart disease can be reversed! That's the definitive answer, I am glad to say.

It's crucial, though, to understand what "reversing" heart disease means. This requires an understanding of heart disease itself — what it is and how it begins.

Cholesterol is widely known as the villain of the heart disease story. This may surprise you, but your body actually needs a healthy amount of cholesterol. It's an essential nutrient that the body uses to build cells and hormones. In fact, cholesterol makes up more than half of each cell, maintaining the cell wall's permeability as it protects the cell's core. Cholesterol even provides the body with Vitamin D when broken down by sunlight.

This natural ally of the body can become its enemy, unfortunately, as a result of the way we eat and because of our decreased activity levels.

Healthy children and adults in countries where heart disease is almost unknown have total cholesterol counts of around 118 and 125.

Many adults, particularly in the West, have cholesterol counts that are much higher. They can be so high, in fact, that when a doctor draws the patient's blood, chills it in a test tube, and spins it using a centrifuge, the tube can have a white, fatty layer on top, like cream on top of milk. In the worst cases, the fat makes the entire test tube turn white.

Cholesterol travels through the blood in particles. These particles are much like the globules that form in a frying pan when you are trying to wash out fat after frying bacon. The smaller and denser these particles are, the more damage they can do, because a smaller size allows them to embed more easily in the artery wall.

That's why LDL cholesterol is often called the "bad cholesterol," while HDL cholesterol is known as the "good cholesterol." By its nature, LDL has more power to embed in the arteries than does HDL cholesterol. Ideally, both LDL cholesterol and HDL cholesterol travel as bigger particles and in less dense packets.

Let's discuss density: Imagine throwing a beach ball around a room. The ball bounces around harmlessly. Even if it hits a lamp it's unlikely to do much damage because it has so little density; that is, it carries very little weight for its size.

Now picture a handful of BBs — which are much smaller and denser — being thrown around a room. They'll likely cause havoc, cracking the ceiling, rattling around in the air ducts, exploding light bulbs, and working themselves down into the carpet, where you'll have to dig them out with your fingers. They'll go everywhere and stay there.

Arteries, meanwhile, are made up of millions of individual cells that are aligned at what cardiologists call "tight junctions." This structure allows for elasticity; the artery can dilate, or stretch to get larger, and also constrict, becoming smaller. Each artery is like a balloon in this way. Being made this way lets the artery accommodate changes in blood pressure, like when your heart pumps faster during exercise, or more slowly during sleep.

Even Mild High Blood Pressure Is a 'Silent Killer'

Constant hypertension, commonly called high blood pressure, wears out an artery's capacity to stretch and, like a balloon that's been blown up too many times, the lining of the artery becomes less elastic and ruptures more easily.

Because high blood pressure has constantly stretched the artery beyond its natural capacity, arterial cells are no longer as tight. Small, dense particles of cholesterol can easily embed themselves in these "tight junctions." Arteries that have been damaged by high blood pressure can also rupture, causing an aneurysm and internal bleeding into the surrounding tissues.

High blood pressure doesn't cause any perceptible symptoms until the condition has become severe. But even mild high blood pressure constantly damages your arteries. That's why it's called the "silent killer."

As a result of my genetic inheritance from my father, I have to fight high blood pressure. My hypertension never showed up during my regular check ups — that's how insidious it can be. However, when I was working under pressure, a frequent part of my job as a doctor, my borderline normal blood pressure became distinctly abnormal. I had no idea about this until I found myself in the hospital with a major blockage of the main coronary artery leading to the heart.

Other inflammatory conditions, such as rheumatoid arthritis, pneumonia, even common infections, can cause inflammation in the arteries. That inflammation allows particles of cholesterol to embed in the lining at areas that are inflamed, or damaged. A vicious cycle sets in: Embedding of cholesterol leads to more inflammation, and inflammation leads to more embedding of the damaging cholesterol particle.

Cholesterol that embeds in the lining causes inflammation, which attracts white blood cells to the site, leading to the development and progression of atherosclerosis, or hardening of the arteries. This complex process is how cholesterol forms deposits called plaque. The formation of plaque in the arteries is what's known as atherosclerosis.

People react differently to the embedding of cholesterol in the artery's lining, just as they react differently to getting a splinter under the skin. Some people handle splinters easily. They experience only minor irritation as the body repairs the damage. Other people who get splinters, however, can experience significant swelling and become infected.

For one person, the embedding of cholesterol in the artery's lining can be a minor thing that happens all the time with no great damage done. For another person, though, it can be the beginning of catastrophe. It all depends on how the person's body reacts to these tiny, yet insistent, attacks on the artery. Reaction usually depends on the frequency of the damage, a person's general health, and other factors.

Relatively new plaque deposits initiate a process that's much like the formation of a blister. Burn yourself accidently with a clothing iron or on the stove and the spot where you touched the hot surface will become red, signaling damage to the tissues. Soon, a blister will form as the body tries to repair the damage. A plaque deposit is like that blister. The artery lining has been slightly damaged by cholesterol embedding in the wall and an inflammatory condition develops.

As I have noted, inflammation in the arteries also can develop as a result of inflammatory conditions elsewhere in the body, such as rheumatoid arthritis, pneumonia, and various forms of infection. In this case, the inflammation itself can be the factor that attracts cholesterol to the site and results in a buildup of plaque.

Deposits of plaque are also like blisters in that they have liquid centers. Plaque deposits thus are weakest around their edges, where the wall of the plaque is the thinnest. Most of the time, if left alone, they are simply reabsorbed by the body. But they can also rupture, releasing their liquid into the blood stream.

The body reacts to the rupture of a plaque deposit like it reacts to a bleeding wound: It marshals its forces to repair the damage. Sometimes the rupture of a plaque deposit will result in the body's defense mechanisms going haywire. A blood clot can form at the site and cause a heart attack, or this clot can detach and travel through the circulatory system, causing a blockage in the arteries leading to other areas of the heart or other organs.

This is how a heart attack, technically called a myocardial infarction, most commonly occurs: A blood clot delivers a devastating blow to the cardiovascular system. (Blood clots also cause brain-damaging strokes). The clot retards the flow of blood to or within the heart and heart tissue, which rapidly begins to die from lack of oxygen and nutrients. Normal blood flow must be restored as quickly as possible in order to minimize the damage and prevent death.

Luckily, most plaque deposits do not initiate the catastrophic chain of events that lead to heart attacks and strokes. The body successfully copes with these blister-like structures and turns them into fibrotic and calcified deposits. Old plaque becomes as hard as mortar between bricks.

In this state, old, hardened plaques cannot be removed from the arteries by any presently known method other than surgery. Usually, this is unnecessary. Unless an artery has been narrowed by more than 75 percent, blood flow remains largely unaffected.

Free Blood Flow is Crucial to Heart Health

Think of blood flow like traffic on a highway. On a four-lane highway, one lane can be blocked off with little effect on how fast the traffic moves. If two lanes are blocked off, traffic may become heavy but still move along at an optimum rate. Block off three lanes, though, and heavy traffic turns into stop-and-go traffic. The highway turns into a parking lot.

That's what happens in the arteries as well. A lot of plaque deposits can form in the arteries without significantly affecting blood flow.

But if the arteries narrow by 75 percent or more the person is likely to experience angina — they lose their breath easily and can suffer left arm, jaw, and chest pain.

This is a condition that can be managed as long as the plaque build up causing the problems is stable. Early, non-critical, or unstable plaque build ups are the ones we worry about most because these are responsible for heart attacks and strokes. These newer buildups of plaque are also the ones that can actually be removed or eliminated through lifestyle changes in diet and exercise.

A relatively minor reduction in plaque deposits — say 8 percent within the body — can result in major health improvements. This is because eliminating the young deposits of plaque is like opening another lane on the highway. Suddenly, the traffic changes from stop-and-go into moving along again at a good rate.

If you remember nothing else, remember this: A minor reversal in heart disease (the removal of young plaque deposits from the arteries) results in a major improvement in health.

The treatment of heart disease involves the elimination of the several factors that together produce the condition. I treat patients a little differently according to their basic condition. Many times patients have already experienced a "cardiac event." They've had a heart attack, an episode of angina, or they've experienced an arterial blockage that's been treated through angioplasty, a procedure that enlarges the artery by expanding a balloon within it, or the insertion of a stent, a steel mesh tube sometimes coated with drugs that keeps the artery open.

We also see patients who have known risk factors for heart disease: hypertension (high blood pressure), hypercholesterolemia (high cholesterol), hyperglycemia (high blood sugar), weight gain, insulin intolerance, or metabolic syndrome. In these cases, the treatment can be less aggressive but it essentially follows the same course.

For those who have had cardiac events, I tell them that we are in a war and we are going to use every weapon we have to win the war and walk in victory.

The most powerful weapon, always, is recruiting the body's resources as our ally. As all good doctors know, the practice of medicine depends mostly on creating conditions in which the body's own natural ability to heal itself can function most effectively. This is particularly true with heart disease because it only develops and advances when the body's own healing capacities are overwhelmed by a person's bad habits.

For a patient with high cholesterol, in most instances I will pre-scribe a statin drug immediately to get the patient to the target goal. Statins have become controversial, and they can have negative side effects. Once you realize, though, how high cholesterol drives heart disease, you can see how important it is to control cholesterol.

Eventually, I like to discontinue the statin medication, but I want to use it as long as necessary in order to shut down the engine of heart disease.

Statins not only lower high cholesterol but they also have oth-er positive effects. They have anti-inflammatory properties, elimi-nating "free radicals," which are atoms or molecules that can cause destructive chain reactions within a cell. And they are vasodilators as well — that is, they help arteries open up. Usually, when people understand the positive effects of statins they become more accept-ing of their use.

I also typically prescribe fish oil for additional regulation of fat in the blood, low-dose aspirin for its anti-coagulant effect, and other medications as needed.

The patient needs to exercise regularly. I ask my patients to make use of a cardiac rehab facility for supervised exercise three times per week. On his or her "off" days, I want the patient to walk for an hour.

I also put the patient on my heart disease reversal diet. This is a largely plant-based diet, with plenty of fresh fruits and vegetables, whole grains, and — particularly at the beginning — as little fat as possible.

That's because I want the body to go after the fat that's already stored in a patient's cells and fat deposits within the arteries and ev-erywhere else it may be located. If the patient takes fat out of his or her diet, the body will quickly begin using the person's stored up fat reserves for energy. It's the body's version of spring cleaning!

This is perhaps the most important thing of all: We want to see the patient once a month for the first six months and every two months during the next six months. These visits are all-important in the edu-cation process that must go on if the patient is going to successfully implement the recommended changes in his or her life.

The habits of eating fatty foods and getting little exercise are usu-ally ones that a patient has developed over the course of years and years. Reversing these habits is difficult — even with one's life on the line! In fact, I rarely see a patient who is able to make changes immediately and continue with them for long without a system of accountability. Regular visits with the doctor are crucial to keeping patients on track.

Lifestyle changes can gather momentum. The more a person implements the recommended changes, the better he or she feels. This positive feedback promotes additional change.

Heart Disease Can Be Reversed

The good news is that heart disease can be reversed.

It can be done. I'm living proof. My motto is simple: A minor reversal in heart disease results in a major improvement in health.

The first step is reeducation. Anyone who visits a cardiologist already has a baseline concern. Either the person has had a "cardiac event" — a heart attack, stroke, an episode of angina — or the person has been referred by a personal physician because of risk factors.

You need to be absolutely honest with your doctor about what brings you to him or her. In every case, I recommend that the patient come in with his or her spouse or family member — the person who knows you best. A spouse, I find, often remembers symptoms that the patient forgets because of the stress of the situation.

I work up a full family history and do a physical exam. I interview my patient about his or her work environment, trying to determine how much stress the person may be under.

Then I order a full lab workup — Cholesterol counts, triglycerides, markers related to renal and thyroid function, homocysteine, C-reactive protein — the works.

Patients generally take a stress test, either a regular EKG stress test (walking on a treadmill) or a nuclear stress test, in which radioisotopes are introduced into their bloodstream. A nuclear test allows us to see the blood flow as well as track the heart's rhythm.

The amount of time a patient can spend on a treadmill is remarkably predictive of their near-term prognosis. If a patient can spend 10 minutes on a treadmill that's being gradually elevated, the incidence of a fatal myocardial infarction (heart attack) over the next year is likely close to zero.

We do an echo cardiogram to establish the size of the heart and check for murmurs. We perform a carotid ultrasound to look at the thickness of the artery and specifically the intima — the lining of the artery. The carotid artery is often a window to what is happening in the heart and the rest of the circulatory system; the thicker the carotid artery, the greater the underlying disease.

Why am I telling you all this? Because it's the start of the reeducation process, the first and most important step in the battle against heart disease. You will be far more prone to listen to the doctor's advice if the tests he cites are meaningful to you.

Your doctor should guide you along this path by seeing you regularly. I want to see my patients once a month for the first six months, then once every two months for the next six months, then three times the following year.

If your doctor thinks such a schedule is overkill, consider changing physicians. "See me in six months" doesn't work in the battle against heart disease. Believe me.

Counseling is imperative because a cardiac patient goes through an often predictable cycle. At first, he is willing to do just about anything. Over time, though, the patient's resistance to change inevitably increases. Unless your doctor is in front of you on a regular basis, your odds of beating heart disease alone are poor.

Hitting Initial Heart-Healthy Targets

In consultation with your doctor, you should establish and understand the following targets for beating heart disease. The numbers are important, but they will be much more useful if you understand the reasoning behind them. My general targets are:

- Blood pressure of 120/80
- Total cholesterol count under 150
- HDL cholesterol should be greater than 45
- LDL cholesterol should be less than 70
- The particle number for LDL should be less than 1,000
- LDL should be described as "Pattern A," meaning your LDL cholesterol particles are large and buoyant
- Triglyceride count less than 150
- A fasting glucose, serum (sugar) count between 65 and 99
- Body mass index (BMI), the percentage of body weight that comes from fat, should be under 25
- Thyroid, C-reactive protein, and homocysteine all within the normal range

I try as soon as possible to start using natural substances. Niacin (vitamin B3) is terrific at lowering LDL and boosting HDL. Most significantly, it changes dense, small LDL particles into larger, more buoyant particles that do not embed as easily in arterial lining.

Niacin has the unhappy side effect of causing flushing — an uncomfortable rush of blood to the face. This feels like breaking out in a sudden heat rash: hot and prickly. For this reason, the patient needs to start with a low dose of niacin, 250 mg, and build up the amount slowly.

The dosage should be increased by 250 mg every three months. It's best to take the dose at night with aspirin, which mitigates the flushing. If you are asleep and experience minor flushing you probably won't even wake up.

It usually takes a patient one to two years to arrive at the maximum dosage that can be tolerated. Ideally, I'd like to see a patient take from 1,500 to 3,000 mg of niacin daily, but few can reach this level. Any dosage the patient tolerates is a plus.

Fish oils (omega-3 and -6 fatty acids) can provide exceptional benefits to patients who have trouble controlling their triglycerides (another form of fat in the blood). Fish such as salmon, trout, mackerel, and sardines contain large amounts of these fatty acids. For those who want to make sure they get enough fish oil by taking supplements, I recommend 2 grams daily. Some doctors recommend as much as 4 grams.

Fish oils are commonly sold in IU units, so you'll have to consult the label or ask your provider how many IU units translate into 2 grams. (IU units are based on effect, not weight, and so the number of units in a substance varies with the substance.)

There are also common foods and substances that help reduce cholesterol. It's important to realize, though, that each of these has only a marginal effect. They have nothing like the potency of statin drugs. They should be used only once the patient's cholesterol is well under control.

Oat bran and oatmeal are good. I start each day with a bowl of cooked oat bran with blueberries. I put a little maple syrup and nutmeg and cinnamon on top. I prefer this concoction cold and will boil up a batch and save it in the refrigerator for the next two to three days.

Oat bran and oatmeal work like this: They both bind cholesterol in the small intestine, causing the system to eliminate it rather than reabsorb it into the liver. Red rice yeast has effects similar to statins. It's hard to know, though, whether you are getting the real thing or a counterfeit. Some Chinese producers were found to be heightening its statin-like effects by adding a statin into the mix. Be sure you are buying from a reliable provider.

Garlic and vitamin C supplementation also can provide some minor benefit.

Then, I consider medications to treat high blood pressure. I often wait three months, until a patient's hypertension is no longer acute, to see how much improvement can be brought about through diet and exercise. Losing 10 pounds works as well as or better than a typical dose of a blood pressure medication, for instance.

If the patient's blood pressure demands it, through, I usually begin slowly with a once-a-day medication, typically an ACE inhibitor, such as Lisinopril. Over time I may add two more, a beta blocker and a medication from the class of drugs called ARBs. There are other types of blood pressure medications to consider as well.

Along with these prescriptions, I ask the patient to cut out stimulants, such as caffeine and alcohol and to reduce salt intake drastically. Cutting the amount of salt consumed demands more than putting down the shaker. Processed foods are loaded with salt. Freshly cooked meals from a diet that's plant-based are a must.

For patients who have had cardiac events or have been diagnosed with underlying heart disease I prescribe a radical, six-month, plant-based, oil-free diet. This diet concentrates on eating whole grains, potatoes and other starches, legumes (beans), vegetables, and fruit. I'll expand on the ideal diet later.

The patient and his spouse must prepare to implement it by studying what you can eat, clearing the house of junk food and restocking the larder with plenty of good food. It's important that you not become too hungry, that you eat good but modest meals three times a day and choose only healthy snacks.

Most patients find my plant-based diet the toughest part to accept of the seven-step plan to reverse heart disease. It works, though. And you have to adhere to it strictly for only six months. Isn't your life worth a six-month change in your eating pattern?

Ideally, I'd like my patients to restrict themselves to 1,800 calories per day. A plant-based diet makes this easy, as you can eat a lot of food if you cut out dairy, sugar, and oils, which have high calorie counts.

Can You Change Your Life? You'd Better . . .

Next comes stress.

The first key to stress reduction is to realize where you are in life. Most people who are concerned about heart disease are over 50. Women start to go through menopause, and men go through their own version of "the change," often called male menopause.

In both cases, hormones decline: estrogen in women; testosterone in men. (Testosterone also declines in women, and the declines have an impact on libido in both sexes.)

As a result of these hormonal changes, the fuel that drives the engine of cholesterol control runs low. Muscle mass decreases. These changes often lead to weight gain. Additional pounds and our sedentary lifestyle exacerbate muscle loss — a vicious cycle sets in.

People over 50 simply cannot "bounce back" from overwork or stressful situations as well as younger folks. You have to begin to adjust your schedule because you cannot go at the same pace you once did.

When I played middle linebacker, for instance, I could pick up the front end of a Volkswagen. I can't anymore, and I don't expect to be able to for the rest of my life.

Even if you don't suffer from the delusion of invincibility you once had, you might find it hard to think of the ways your schedule might be changed to cut stress. Some years ago, former President Bill Clinton had two stents inserted in his heart. His staff spoke of "trimming his schedule around the edges." But they had to do more than that.

Once again, I find that spouses are my greatest allies in helping their mates implement stress reduction. I often ask couples to go away for a long weekend together and make a list of the ways the patient can alter his (or her) lifestyle. A spouse can usually point out how late the patient stays at work, for example. Spouses can also be more candid about a patient's drinking and smoking habits.

In my own case, I had to give up working until 11:30 p.m. every day. I had to come home at dinnertime in order to have a decent, modest meal, instead of waiting until I was famished then vacuuming up cafeteria food. Working shorter hours decreased my income, but that was a necessary adjustment as part of my recovery program.

You must realize that you need a balance in your life between work and recreation. You need to draw closer to your family members and spend more time talking to them. Talking to your spouse is the No. 1 stress reducer and, for most, the easiest to implement.

Take time — dedicated time — to pray. Concentrate on all the things for which you are grateful. It is impossible to feel stressed when you are feeling grateful. It's literally impossible: the two emotions are polar opposites.

Stressful events inevitably will come to every person and household. But if you modify your schedule appropriately, you'll be able to handle it better.

The Ultimate Change Is Finding New Purpose

Leisure cannot be an end in itself. It's better understood as "re-creation," a time of putting yourself back together in order to return to work. That doesn't necessarily mean slaving away at a stressful, high-powered job. It means working at an appropriate pace for where you are in life.

I tell my patients that I don't want them to retire — ever. You sit down in that recliner and you start to rot and decay. Get up and move! You've probably acquired tremendous skills over your lifetime, and these should be employed for others' benefit. Don't waste your life and your talents by being sick.

As you do this, you'll discover that life and human history are not a competition but something of far greater gravity. Life is a war, with a good side and a bad side.

Take action on behalf of the good side and you'll quickly see where the lines are drawn. And God, whatever you might have thought previously, will become real to you. I guarantee it.

CHAPTER 18

Fight Heart Disease with Dr. Crandall's Life Plan Diet

When I have occasion to discuss diet with a patient, he or she is usually eager to listen because they have recently experienced a heart attack or another traumatic cardiac event. Often, the patient and spouse sit in my office, their faces drained of color, wondering if there's hope. My message: There's not only hope, but the real possibility of completely eliminating heart disease as a health threat.

Most patients can hardly believe that such good news can be true, and are ready to leap tall buildings in order to realize this possibility. At least at first.

Our instinct to survive is a powerful motivator.

The way we live — our schedules, our jobs, and our relationships with family, friends, and community — largely rules how we eat. It has been that way throughout human civilization. And the truth is that almost every "diet" works. Not all are heart healthy, but most diet plans, if you abide by them, will help you lose weight.

But the opposite is also true: Diets don't work. Because unless we fundamentally change the way we live, our long-term habits will eventually reemerge and trump any dietary restrictions we try to impose on ourselves.

There will come a day when we're tired, bored, unhappy, or at our wits' end — and then Ben and Jerry turn us back into Chunky Monkeys.

Throughout my life I've had two great interests: medicine and anthropology. I've traveled the world to study ancient and contemporary cultures, and have learned to look at health as a culturally driven feature of human life. I have also learned that heart disease is a cultural phenomenon that is distinct to the modern Western lifestyle.

Other cultures simply do not suffer from heart disease as much as Americans. This stands as compelling evidence that heart disease is the product of the way we live and eat.

This fact was brought to wide public attention through the 2005 publication of *The China Study* by T. Colin Campbell and Thomas M. Campbell. This book reported on the health and nutritional practices among men in 65 rural Chinese counties where the population ate a largely plant-based diet. The authors found that death rates from heart disease among the sample Chinese population were 17 times lower than American men. And even though the rural Chinese men consumed more calories per kilogram than Americans, their body weight remained 20 percent lower.

The Campbells' findings on nutrition and diet offer important insights on how we think about health and the Western lifestyle. The present epidemics of heart disease, Type 2 diabetes, and even certain types of cancer are the product of widespread affluence in the post-industrial age. We are addicted to living on starches, sugars, fatty meats, and salt, and sitting in front of the television as we consume them.

Many people are taking these findings to heart. There's a whole movement — often called the Caveman Diet or the Stonehenge Diet — that encourages people to eat as ancient man did before agriculture set in and large grain crops started being produced.

Hunter-gatherer societies still exist, of course, at the fringes of civilization. They still live off the fruits of local flora and the root vegetables on the ground. They still catch and kill fish and wild game.

There's a wealth of evidence that hunter-gatherer societies, both ancient and modern, exhibit remarkably low incidences of heart disease, Type 2 diabetes, arthritis, and dementia. Some have suggested that if we tailor our diet to that of the hunter-gatherer societies, we would find ourselves similarly free of the diseases that plague us.

The ultimate case in point comes from my patients who are 100 years old and older. I have many in my care now, and every single one lives the same way. My centenarians are active: They garden, write poetry, paint, do chores around the house, and take walks. They live highly regimented lives, waking up at the same time every day, going to bed at the same time each night, and even eat the same foods every day.

They will have an egg, a piece of whole wheat toast, and a piece of fruit for breakfast. At lunch, they'll eat a small salad and a bowl of soup. At dinner, more vegetables, a starch such as potatoes or rice, and a small portion of meat.

They never overeat and rarely snack. They have disciplined themselves to eat small portions, eating to live rather than living to eat.

That's the way you live to be 100.

Plant-Based Diets Treat Heart Disease

It's long been known that eating right can prevent heart disease and related problems such as Type 2 diabetes. What fewer people know is that with proper diet, heart disease can even be reversed. The percentage of obstruction in the vessels can actually be brought down. It takes only a small improvement to make a major difference in blood flow.

Dr. Dean Ornish and Dr. Caldwell Esselstyn have been among the leaders in showing that a plant-based diet can bring about an improvement in over 82 percent of patients with heart disease.

Just what is a plant-based diet? It's a diet concentrated on raw and cooked vegetables of every description, along with fresh fruit, whole grains, and legumes (beans). Dr. Esselstyn excludes red meat, chicken, fish, dairy, and oils from his plant-based diet.

Dr. Ornish allows for egg whites and nonfat dairy products. He also makes a distinction between what he calls the "Reversal Diet," which strictly excludes meat products, and his "Prevention Diet" that allows for modifications.

While I have tremendous respect for the work that Drs. Ornish and Esselstyn have done, I have come to believe that a strictly plant-based diet is not the best choice for many people. Let me say quickly that if you have serious cardiovascular disease, it is absolutely the way to begin, and may be necessary indefinitely.

At my medical practice in Palm Beach, Fla., we run a "Metabolic Clinic" for patients who have suffered a cardiac event. All such patients are advised to go on a radical, plant-based diet and stay on it until they hit a series of weight and blood profile targets. However, once those targets have been hit, the strict plant-based diet can be moderated to include a more well-rounded diet.

Dr. Crandall's Life Plan Diet

There is now evidence to suggest that what people often call the "Mediterranean Diet" is even better than the plant-based diet for maintaining long-term heart health. The Mediterranean diet is also easier to follow for years on end. The inclusion of Greek-style yogurt, olives, garlic, goat cheese, and the occasional glass of red wine provide variety and pleasure that make the diet more accommodating to epicurean tastes.

"Dr. Crandall's Life Plan Diet" incorporates aspects of the Ornish/Esselstyn plant-based diet along with features of the Mediterranean diet. It avoids the pitfalls of Ornish/Esselstyn in recommending too much starch (which can lead to weight gain) and too little protein.

Of course, I'd like to be able to tell you that my diet contains some secret formula that no one has ever thought of before, bringing about a complete revolution in nutritional thinking.

But, like most true things, my diet's wisdom is based on ideas that have been understood for ages. Much of it as simple as what your mother told you: Eat your fruits and vegetables.

In fact, you should fill up on fruits and vegetables before anything else, because one of the amazing things about fruits and vegetables is that you positively cannot stuff yourself with them. Unlike grains and meat, fruits and vegetables send a clear signal to your brain that you are full, and it's time to stop eating.

Over a period of two weeks to a month, if you eat fruits and vegetables and little else, you'll find the urge to stuff yourself going away. That won't happen if you lard up your potatoes with butter; it will if you just eat the potato.

You can add small amounts of olive oil to your salads. People have been thriving for millennia on olive oil. It has tremendous antioxidant and healing properties.

When you are "dressing" a salad, remember to keep it skimpy. Use the oil sparingly in a vinaigrette dressing, and put your portion to the side where you can just dip your fork into it as needed.

The major difference between my diet and Ornish and Esselstyn involves protein. Yes, it is possible to get protein from non-animal sources like nuts and beans of all varieties. A diet that allows for goat cheese and nonfat hard cheeses contains an additional source of protein as well.

But there is a real role for animal-based proteins in any diet. After all, human beings have been fishing and hunting wild game for eons. Today, we have to be more cautious about the meats we eat because the way we get our food has changed so much.

In times past, red meats were reserved for special occasions, such as a wedding feast. Not only that, ancient people didn't have cows raised on antibiotic-laced feed or hormonally plumped lamb chops.

Red meat should be avoided except on special occasions, and even chicken should be consumed in small portions. Because red meats should be an infrequent part of your diet, try to restrict your red meat to wild game like bison and venison.

I recommend that most of your animal-based proteins come from fish. Fatty fish are rich in omega-3 oils; leaner fish are nutrient-rich without being high in calories.

My Timetable for a Healthy Diet

- **6:00 a.m.** I kick-start my metabolism with a glass of water with lemon, then I go for an hour-long walk to get my blood flowing. Fresh air and gentle, moderate exercise help get the day started.

- **7:00 a.m.** When I come home, I have a breakfast of three egg whites and one egg yolk, sliced cucumber, sliced tomatoes, steamed spinach, one piece of whole-grain toast with a little orange marmalade, and a cup of coffee. Whole grains are digested more slowly and evenly when they are combined with protein. Eggs even out the insulin production, and keep me feeling satisfied and energetic much longer.

Not so long ago, I was eating only oatmeal and fruit in the morning, just as the Ornish plan recommends. However, I found that I ran out of energy at about 10 o'clock each morning. Even whole-grain starches cause a pronounced rise in the secretion of insulin, which eventually leads to a sudden drop in blood sugar.

- **12:00 p.m.** For lunch, I have a salad with a strip of chicken or fish. I use very little dressing and always place it on the side. Once again, the protein helps the meal carry me through the afternoon. For variety, I'll make myself a sandwich of hard cheese, avocado, and sliced turkey on whole-wheat bread.

- **2:30 p.m.** A handful of raw walnuts or almonds helps me get through a hungry spell in the mid-afternoon. I always have some nearby, just in case. If I get really hungry, I'll complement the nuts with an apple.

- **6:00 p.m.** For dinner, I have fish, steamed vegetables, and a bowl of fruit for dessert.

- Every once in a while I'll have a piece of dark chocolate as a healthy indulgence.

I eat like this every day, especially during the work week. On the weekend, my wife and I allow ourselves a little variety to keep the diet from feeling like a burden. That's OK as long as you go right back to the plan and stay with it.

In sum, keep it simple, keep it light, and keep it fresh. Find healthy foods that you enjoy, and explore the whole world of seasonings that can make healthy meals like this into real taste treats.

Many people ask how they can implement such a diet gradually. The truth is, you can't. You have to challenge yourself head-on. Throw out all the junk in your house, go shopping with a completely altered shopping list, and learn how to cook tasty, healthy meals from the foods I've recommended.

The other day, a somewhat famous person came into my office. He was the brother of a big movie star, and he was accustomed to living the high life, eating and drinking whatever he wanted, whenever he wanted. The result: He had a massive anterior wall heart attack. His blood pressure and cholesterol were elevated; he was overweight and inactive.

He sat in my office with his wife, and I gave him the good news — that heart disease can be reversed — and the bad news — that it was going to require a complete change in his lifestyle.

The man and his wife both balked. They enjoyed their lifestyle — or claimed they did — and didn't see the point in living if they couldn't indulge in their customary pleasures. They left my office without taking any of my advice, and now my one-time patient is likely on his way to a premature end.

At least they were honest. Many people I see in my office believe the exact same thing, but the fear engendered by a cardiac event masks those sentiments — for a while. Once they start feeling better, their addiction to indulgence resurfaces. They quit their diets and don't want to talk to their doctors anymore — until the next cardiac event.

Such attitudes are one reason physicians do little more than pre-scribe drugs. Doctors don't want to take the time to educate patients because so few patients are willing to comply with their advice. It's easier to control what medications the patient takes, and so doctors are content to control what they can.

The Most Powerful Motivator: Love

With patients who have a strong religious faith, I often feel I can speak more freely. I remind them that their lives ultimately belong to God, who made them for a greater purpose than mere indulgence. All of us were put on this Earth to love our families, our neighbors, and even our enemies. We can't do that properly if we are sick, and bad eating habits are one of the main causes of sickness in this country.

The Apostle Paul writes to the church in Rome: "For the kingdom of God is not a matter of eating and drinking, but of righteousness, peace, and joy in the Holy Spirit."

Even if you are not a person of faith, you should be able to see that implementing the diet and lifestyle changes necessary to beating heart disease is ultimately a matter of what you value. Fear of death can only motivate you for a little while. In the end, it's what you truly love that will determine whether or not you take the steps to successfully fight heart disease. That is the most powerful motivator in the world.

Do you love eating and drinking more than your family? More than what you might yet accomplish in your life? Have you given up, or do you want to live?

If you start eating as I've recommended, you'll feel so much better that you'll rediscover the joys in life. Eat right in order to live a life that's truly worth living — that's my life-plan diet.

CHAPTER 19

7 Super Foods for Your Heart

Here's a daunting proposition: Whether you know it or not, every time you eat something, you are making a conscious choice about your heart health. Will that food you are consuming make your heart healthier or will it contribute to conditions that may lead to a heart attack?

This may seem like an exaggeration, but it's not. Just look at the statistics — heart disease is the No. 1 killer of men *and* women in America. That death rate is directly linked to high blood levels of cholesterol, the substance that gums up your coronary arteries and leads to heart attacks. And high levels of cholesterol are linked directly to what we choose to eat.

I learned this lesson myself in 2002, when I ended up in the emergency room — not in my usual role of Chief of Cardiology, but as a patient. I'd come close to having a heart attack, thanks to a blockage in my left coronary artery, and the doctor had performed an angioplasty and inserted a stent to restore the blood flow.

At that time, my doctor also informed me I had developed a smaller blockage on the right side of my heart. This blockage would also eventually require surgery.

"No more surgery," I told him firmly. "I'm going to take care of this myself."

My doctor was skeptical. But I revamped my diet and saw my cholesterol fall from 200 to 128, the ultra-low level found in cultures where heart disease is nonexistent.

A large part of my success came from the 7 "super" foods that I included in my diet. These foods will supercharge your heart and lower your cholesterol, and can even reverse coronary artery disease.

And there are other benefits that you can reap from including these super foods in your diet, including:

• Losing weight
• Preventing diabetes
• Strengthening your immune system
• Blocking cellular changes that can lead to cancer

But don't think that I'm asking you to give up the pleasure of eating in order to improve your heart health. Not at all. Because not only are these super foods super-healthy, they are also flavorful and versatile, offering many different ways to enjoy them. So there's absolutely no reason why these super foods shouldn't make an appearance at your table every day.

Here's a rundown of 7 super, heart-healthy foods, as well as an explanation of why each one is so good for you.

1. Blueberries Stand Out From the Bunch

Many different kinds of berries — including blackberries, strawberries, and raspberries — offer a wide array of health benefits. But without question, blueberries are the standout in the bunch.

Blueberries are low in calories, with just 80 calories per cup, and contain no fat. They help keep the heart's blood vessels healthy, and also provide the body with fiber — which helps lower cholesterol.

They are also loaded with minerals, including manganese, which plays an important part in bone development and helps to convert protein, carbohydrates and fat into energy.

But where blueberries really excel is in their antioxidant power. How rich in antioxidants are blueberries? The United States Department of Agriculture (USDA) recently rated 100 foods on their antioxidant power, and blueberries received an "A" rating. They also suppress inflammation, which is a key driver of coronary artery disease.

One of the questions I get asked most often is if blueberries retain their health benefits when they are not eaten fresh. The good news is that it doesn't matter if blueberries are fresh, frozen, dried, or cooked.

In fact, no matter how they are prepared, the nutrients in blueberries remain some of the most healthful things you can eat.

2. Oatmeal Is the Best Defense Against Cholesterol

You may already know that oatmeal helps lower cholesterol. But you may not realize just how good a job it does. It's a fact: No matter what health organization is doing the test, whenever the subject turns to cholesterol-lowering foods, oatmeal tops the list.

Studies published by the *Journal of the American Medical Association* and the *American Journal of Clinical Nutrition* have shown that eating oatmeal regularly lowers "bad" LDL cholesterol just as well as drug therapy.

But that's not all; in addition to lowering cholesterol, eating oatmeal lowers blood pressure and may help prevent diabetes.

And oatmeal is not only good for your heart. Like most of the other foods on this list, oatmeal ranks low on the glycemic index, which is good news for people with diabetes.

Hot oatmeal is a great way to start the day, but there are also other ways to get your daily dose of oats. You can substitute oat flour for wheat flour in recipes, or use it instead of bread crumbs when baking fish.

3. Almonds Contain Good Fat

In some cultures, almonds are symbols of hope or good fortune. That actually seems appropriate, as we now know that they lead to good heart health as well.

Eating just a handful of almonds each day has been found to lower LDL cholesterol by as much as 9 percent.

In addition to lowering cholesterol, almonds are loaded with the antioxidant vitamin E and essential minerals such as:
- Calcium
- Iron
- Magnesium
- Phosphorus
- Potassium
- Zinc

They also contain omega-3 fatty acids, fiber, and protein.

But perhaps the best thing about almonds is that even though they may taste fattening, they actually contain the "good" monounsaturated oils, not the nasty saturated stuff. So they can fill you up without getting you fat.

Like oat flour, almond flour can also be substituted as a healthier alternative to refined white (wheat) flour when baking.

4. Salmon: The Star Among Fish

I recently read a news account about a Vietnamese woman who has lived to the age of 121. The article noted that she dines only on fish and rice.

In fact, her diet comes as no surprise to me, as studies consistently find that people who frequently eat fish live longer than those who don't.

While many types of fish can be part of a healthy diet, the star among them is salmon. Rich in omega-3 fatty acids, salmon offers many benefits, including helping prevent heart attack and stroke, reducing high blood pressure, and normalizing glucose levels.

Salmon is also rich in vitamin A, riboflavin (vitamin B2), vitamin B6, vitamin B12, and niacin. In addition, salmon contains folate, which works with the B vitamins to help lower levels of the amino acid homocysteine. High levels of homocysteine may be a marker for coronary artery disease risk.

When you're preparing fish, always grill, bake, or pan-fry it (preferably with heart-healthy olive oil). Deep frying salmon takes away its health benefits.

5. Olive Oil Stops Blood Clots

The longevity of people who live in Mediterranean countries — and their low rate of heart disease — has long been attributed to their widespread use of olive oil, which does not contain saturated or trans fats.

Even though it's rich tasting, olive oil is a "good fat," abundant in monounsaturated fatty acids. When you substitute this type of fat for saturated or trans fats like butter or margarine, you reap huge health benefits.

Olive oil can also help lower LDL cholesterol and help prevent blood from clotting in the arteries, which leads to heart attack.

In addition, olive oil may help normalize blood glucose levels. This factor is very beneficial for people who suffer from diabetes.

Although olive oil is healthy, it is also packed with calories, so it should be used sparingly. Sprinkle it on salads with a fork, or use an olive oil spray to coat the frying pan before cooking.

You can even bake with olive oil; generally, what you want to do is substitute three tablespoons of olive oil for a quarter cup of butter.

Olive oil can turn rancid, so it's best to keep it away from light or heat; store it in a cool, dark place, or keep it in the refrigerator. Also, don't pay high prices for extra-virgin olive oil if you are going to use it for cooking. Reserve the high-priced stuff for the olive oil you'll sprinkle on your salad.

6. Legumes Are a Great Meat Substitute

Legumes (beans, peas, and nuts) are one of the best food sources of soluble fiber. Beans, especially, make a great meat substitute because, like meat, they are rich in protein and filling.

However, because beans are also packed with fiber, while meat has none, beans are digested more slowly. This makes you feel full longer and makes it easier to lose weight. In addition, beans can help lower bad cholesterol, and are an excellent source of antioxidants.

In fact, in the USDA study that rated foods on their antioxidant power, three types of beans made the top of the list: small red beans, red kidney beans and pinto beans. Black beans, navy beans, and black eyed peas were high on the list as well.

7. Soymilk Is Rich in Vitamins and Minerals

Rounding out the list of super foods is soymilk, which is made from fresh, mature soybeans.

Soymilk is an especially popular choice among people who are lactose intolerant. However, the healthy ingredients in soymilk offer plenty of benefits that everyone can enjoy.

For instance, soymilk is plant-based, so it's cholesterol free. It also has health benefits that dairy milk does not, including heart-healthy omega-3 fats. Like dairy milk, soymilk contains protein, along with these vitamins and minerals:
- Copper
- Iron
- Manganese
- Niacin
- Riboflavin
- Thiamin
- Vitamin B6

Soymilk also ranks low on the glycemic index, making it a good choice for people with diabetes. Soymilk can be substituted any place that milk is used. Just make sure you choose unsweetened soymilk, as the sugar can really add up.

Some people prefer to change their eating habits drastically and whole-heartedly embrace a plant-based eating plan; others prefer to make changes gradually.

What's important is that you pledge to start eating healthier today, and incorporate these foods into your eating plan, either quickly, or gradually. Whichever way you choose, your heart will thank you for it.

CHAPTER 20

Your 90-Day Plan to Reverse Heart Disease

If you are reading this book, it is most likely you already have heart disease or you are at high risk of developing it. You have gotten into this situation largely due to bad habits. Like most of my new patients, you eat the wrong foods, spend hours in front of the TV or computer, and you also worry about things that are not within your control. You may even still be a smoker. None of this matters now. This is a brand new day! Now that you are reading this book, you have taken the first step in your victory over heart disease and I know you will succeed. To ensure your success, I've developed this unique 90-day plan to get you started.

Week 1 — Start Planning

There is an old saying, "When you don't plan, you plan to fail." This is especially true when it comes to fixing your heart. The key to creating healthy habits is planning for success. After all, you don't start out the day from scratch, facing a myriad of decisions about what to eat, what clothes to wear, or what route to take to work. If you did, you would never get out the door. These habits are engrained in you and they are killing you. My 90-day plan will help you change all that.

By the time you finish this 90-day plan, you will be walking one hour a day. You'll do it like clockwork, even if that sounds daunting now. This week, you will start off by walking 15-minutes each day. When will you do it? Think about your schedule. Then, I want you to lace up your sneakers (or any other comfortable walking shoes) and head out the door. You are already walking away from heart disease (read pages 116-118 for more details).

Also, I want you to start shedding your old eating habits and replacing them with healthy new ones. Most likely, you've tried before, but by the end of this 90-day plan, you will either be at your ideal weight or you will be well on your way. First, though, you must know how overweight you are. To do this, you need to know your Body Mass Index, or BMI. This measurement is very important because it will also show you how much belly fat you have. Belly fat is very dangerous. Learning about it will change the way you look at your body fat forever (read page 5 for more details).

Now let's begin revamping your eating habits. Breakfast is the most important meal of the day, so let's start with that. Get a notebook, or start a food journal on your computer. For seven days, keep track of what you eat for breakfast, and write it down (read page 176 for more details).

By the end of this first week, here are the target goals you should have achieved:

- You are walking 15 minutes a day at least.

- You have calibrated your current BMI and you know the difference between where you are now and the ideal BMI.

- You will understand why eating a good breakfast is important and you will also know what your typical breakfast is like and how to begin making healthy changes.

Week 2 —Plan to Eat Healthy

Now, you will lay the groundwork to begin changing your bad eating habits. Healthy eating does not happen overnight! Following a plant-based, whole food diet is the key, and this is the diet that you will follow for the rest of your life. As you build your new habit, though, you will find that you will enjoy this way of eating, and you will gradually lose your taste for the old, chemical-laden food you used to eat.

So here's your first task for this week — take action! Throw out all your fat-laden, processed foods — you're not going to need them any more. Clear it all out to make room for heart-healthy food! Toss out anything that is packaged, processed and filled with chemicals. This includes chemically-laden, low-fat foods. Now, read about the diet that I enjoy every day. It's also the diet that has lowered my blood pressure, cholesterol, and kept my heart healthy (read pages 137-139 for more details).

Now, let's go shopping for breakfast foods! Take a look at the Simple Heart Cure Food List, and chose your favorite foods for breakfast, along with at least two you plan to try. Then, head for either an organic supermarket, or a supermarket that has a large fresh produce section, as well as organic eggs, nuts and nonfat diary products. If you are reluctant to do this because you've heard organic foods are more expensive, take out a sheet of paper and figure out what you'll be saving once you eliminate junk food, fast food, cigarettes and excess alcohol from your life. You'll be amazed at the savings (read pages 171-174 for details).

Keep up with your walking regimen. Add 15 minutes, so you will be walking 30 minutes each day. Don't forget to chart your progress.

By the end of Week 2 you should have achieved the following:

- Buy a scale. You need to know your weight and the goal weight you need to reach. (In most cases, it will be what you weighed in high school). If you already have a scale, make sure it's accurate. If it's old and rusted, throw it out. Read pages 71-73 for more details.

- You are walking 30 minutes a day at least.

- You have cleared out all of the processed, packaged food from your fridge and cupboards

- You have visited the supermarket and purchased enough food to make three healthy breakfasts.

Week 3 — Revamp Your Breakfast

It's time to start revamping the way you eat, starting with breakfast. Review my Simple Heart Cure Menu Plan and, using the foods that you bought last week, get the ingredients ready for your first week of healthy breakfasts. Also, be sure to include some of the foods that are super-good for your heart. Once you find a breakfast that appeals to you, start eating it every day, or, if you like variety, select two or three, but no more than that. I want you to feel comfortable with your new menu choices before adding more.

Now that you have your breakfast mapped out, it's time to start fixing them. Also, don't forget to write down what you eat in your food journal (read page 150 for more details). Remember, breakfast is only the beginning. You are probably curious to find out how this new, healthy breakfast you are enjoying will fit into the rest of your day, so read all about how I structure my eating on a typical day (read pages 139-140 for more details).

I also want you to feel comfortable with the activity levels you are achieving, so you don't need to add any more walking to your schedule more than that 30-minute walk. But boredom can be the enemy of a daily workout, so try varying your route. Have you found the best time of the day to do it? Do you feel rushed in the morning? Try an evening walk. Experiment.

By the end of Week Three you should have achieved the following:

- You are preparing a healthy breakfast every day.

- You are thinking about revamping your lunch.

- You are enjoying a 30-minute walk and also varying your route to learn which one suits you best.

- Weigh yourself and chart your progress.

Week 4 - Learn Your Risk Factors

Now that you're actually changing your habits, you want to know the reason behind some of these fixes. Over and over in this book, you'll notice that I mention "risk factors." Risk factors are specific conditions that separately increase the probability that you will develop heart disease, or that you will suffer a heart attack. But a simple list of risk factors really means nothing —the only way to figure out your risk factors is to learn which ones pertain to you. Risk factors can also affect you differently depending on your gender (read pages 61-66 for more details).

By knowing your risk factors, you can also tell which of the Heart Health Target Numbers you need to reach. Target numbers include your BMI, cholesterol level, blood pressure, etc. To know where you stand on these numbers, you need to undergo a physical exam with lab tests. If it's been awhile, make an appointment with your doctor and ask for these tests. After all, you can't know how to map a trip unless you know your destination. These numbers will tell you where you stand and where you need to go (read page 130 for more details).

This week, you're adding another 15 minutes on that walk, so you are up to 45 minutes a day. That's terrific! If you hadn't been active before embarking on this 90-day plan, or you were walking less, take a few minutes to really pat yourself on the back!

By the end of Week Four you should have achieved the following:

- Make a list of all the risk factors that pertain to you.

- Make a list of your Target Numbers. Write down where you are, and also what your goal should be. If you don't know your Target Numbers, make an appointment with your doctor to find out.

- You are now walking 45 minutes a day. Congratulations!

- Take a look at your sneakers or walking shoes. Are they wearing out? Shoes are like tires for your feet; check them regularly to find out if they need replacing.

- Weigh yourself and chart your progress.

Week 5: Target High Blood Pressure

Of all the risk factors, high blood pressure is among the deadliest. High blood pressure damages the blood vessels in your heart and brain, aging them prematurely, and setting the stage for cardiovascular disease, which means you are at greater risk for heart disease and stroke. But what's the good news? For the past four weeks, you have steadily taken steps to reduce your blood pressure, so it may already be dropping (read pages 85-92 for more details).

Medication can be a very important part of controlling high blood pressure. By following my 90-day plan, you should be able to reduce, or even eventually eliminate, your medications. In the meantime, though, you must understand why blood pressure medication is so important, how it works, and which are the best (read page 132 for more details).

Also, how is your healthy breakfast coming? Now, go back to your menu plan and follow the same steps you did for breakfast to shop for ingredients and create seven days of healthy lunches. Pay close attention to eliminating the sodium in your food. And remember to keep walking!

By the end of Week Five you should have achieved the following:

- Learn what your blood pressure is and what is your target goal.

- If you are not at your blood pressure goal, discuss a plan with your doctor that will get you there.

- Know if your blood pressure is under controlled and, if not, discuss an action plan with your doctor.

- If your blood pressure is not under control, make sure you are following the directions for each medication to the letter. Purchase a compartmentalized pillbox or make lists or use electronic reminders to stay on track.

- Keep up that 45-minute a day walk. Walking is a key way to lower blood pressure.

- Weigh yourself at least once a week and chart your progress. A weight loss of 10 pounds equals the reduction of one blood pressure medication.

Week 6: Conquer Cholesterol

Another risk factor we'll be targeting in this 90-day plan is cholesterol, so let's get going! Abnormal cholesterol levels are not the only risk factors for heart disease, but they are key. While our bodies manufacture cholesterol naturally, having too much of this substance builds up in the coronary arteries (read pages 124-126 for more details).

Also, learn about the advanced lipid profile. This test tells you the composition of your cholesterol. Small, deadly particles that embed themselves in the coronary arteries and damage the arteries are more dangerous than light, fluffy particles. There are ways to change your cholesterol composition, but you need to know which type you have first (read pages 70-71 for more details).

As with high blood pressure, cholesterol-lowering drugs play a key role in reducing cholesterol, at least in the beginning (read pages 77-84 for more details). As you'll soon learn, though, I believe that patients should be encouraged to get off medication by changing their lifestyle. By adopting a heart-healthy lifestyle, you may be able to reduce, and even eliminate, your need for cholesterol-lowering medication. Cutting out saturated fat is key to achieving this goal and the best way to do that is through diet. So, now that you've replaced your breakfast and lunch with a plant-based diet, you are well on your way to achieving this goal.

By the end of Week Six you should have achieved the following:

- Know what your cholesterol and triglyceride levels are and your target goals.

- Follow the same steps you did to create a healthy plant-based breakfast and lunch to begin planning to add healthy dinners next week

- Add 15 minutes to your 45-minute daily walk. Congratulations — you have achieved a very important milestone on your way to heart health, and you are now walking an hour a day.

- Weigh yourself and chart your progress.

Week 7: Defeat Diabetes

When insulin was discovered in 1922, diabetes changed from an invariably fatal disease that killed within a short time to being thought of as a manageable, chronic disease. This could not be further from the truth —diabetes remains a deadly killer. In fact, having diabetes more than doubles the heart attack risk in men, and triples it in women. This is your week to learn all about diabetes and what you can do to achieve victory over it (read pages 27-34 for more details).

By now, too, you're probably getting more comfortable with my plant-based, whole foods form of eating, so keep trying our recipes and tweaking your preferences by using my menu plan (for more details, read pages 137-139). Also, I want you to keep to that one-hour a day walk, but, by now, you may be ready for some added variety (read page 118 for more details).

By the end of Week Seven you should have achieved the following:

- Know what your glucose status is. Ask your doctor to screen you for diabetes.

- If you have diabetes or pre-diabetes (also known as insulin resistance), discuss a management plan with your doctor.

- If you have either of these conditions, you are at increased risk for heart disease. Talk to your doctor about a plan to monitor you for any sign that heart disease is developing.

- Continue your one-hour daily walk.

- Weigh yourself and chart your progress.

Week 8 — De-Stress Your Life

Stress, which is a key risk factor for heart disease, often doesn't get the respect it deserves. Indeed, I never considered stress that key a factor until it almost caused my own heart attack a decade ago. But now, I'm very aware that, when you're under stress, your body releases dangerous hormones that can elevate your cholesterol levels, raise your blood pressure and damage your heart (read pages 133-134 for details).

Happily, exercise is a terrific stress buster, so, because you've been following my 90-day plan, and you're now walking an hour a day, you're already beating stress (read pages 118-121 for details). In addition, I want to share with you one of the best ways I have personally found to deal with the stress, which is turning to the Lord. Living a faith-based life is a key way to find contentment. I have discussed how to bring faith to your life earlier in this book.

By the end of Week Eight you should have achieved the following:

- Take a "Stress Inventory." Think about your life and areas that might be giving you stress. Jot them down, and look for ways that you can minimize stress.

- If you are under high stress, and you can't think of ways to reduce your stress level, you might consider taking a stress reduction class or confiding in a counselor or a member of the clergy.

- Continue your one-hour daily walk.

- Try out a new recipe this week, or incorporate a different type of food or vegetable that you've never tried before into your menu.

- Weigh yourself and chart your progress. Are you losing weight? If you're not, or your unhappy with your progress, start keeping track of the calories you're consuming. If you cut down to 1,200 calories, you'll find the weight comes off more quickly.

Week 9 — Learn the Warning Signs of a Heart Attack

If you are a heart attack survivor, or if you have coronary artery disease or are at high risk, all of the steps in this 90-day plan will help you toward heart health. Still, it's wise to take precautions, and you can do that by knowing the warning signs of an impending heart attack. It's also imperative that you know what to do in case such warning signs strike (read page 108 for more details).

Remember, if you fit the risk profile for a heart attack, this means you are also at risk for a stroke. Not all strokes are major ones; minor, or temporary strokes can occur. These are called transient ischemic strokes, or TIA's (read pages 38-40 for more details).

Another major risk factor that I haven't discussed with you in depth in this 90-day plan is smoking. If you smoke, this is your week to plan to quit (read pages 8, 37-38, and 40 for more details).

By the end of Week Nine you should have achieved the following:

- Be comfortable shopping for your heart-healthy breakfast, lunch and dinner meal plans. Know how to use recipes, and also experiment with different ingredients, like fruits and vegetables, that you've never tried before.

- Walk an hour a day and do an additional activity twice a week, such as tennis, gardening, or ballroom dancing.

- If you smoke, ask your doctor for smoking cessation advice, including medication. Make sure that you have a definite plan to quit. No more putting it off!

- Weigh yourself and chart your progress.

Week 10 — Get Strong!

Now that you're walking and doing other types of cardiovascular exercise that will strengthen your heart, it's time to build up your muscles. Once, we thought it was normal to lose muscle mass as you age, but now we know that, no matter how old you are, you can gain muscle mass. This will benefit your entire body, including your heart (read page 119 for more details). Also, no matter what your age, your hormones also play an important part in your heart health (read pages 24-25 for more details).

How are you doing on the Simple Heart Cure Menu Plan? By now, you should be enjoying a heart-healthy breakfast and lunch, so it's time to add dinner as well. Check out the suggested menus on pages 176-186. One way to check on how you are doing is to weigh yourself regularly.

By the end of Week Ten you should have achieved the following:

- Added weight training 2-3 times a week to your daily regimen

- Shopped for and planned out your first heart-healthy dinners

- Weighed yourself and charted your progress

Week 11 — Develop Good Sleep Habits

Good heart health depends not only on the habits you follow while you're awake, but also your sleep habits as well. You must get a good night's sleep and, if your not, it's now time to correct it. If you're tired during the day, you may have sleep apnea, a dangerous sleep disorder, which is linked to high blood pressure, cardiovascular disease, and even dementia. The problem, though, is that most people with sleep apnea are unaware of it, which can be tragic, especially because sleep apnea is very fixable (read pages 22-23 for more details).

Another hidden risk factor I want you to attack this week lurks in your mouth! Periodontal disease, which is also known as gum disease, creates an inflammatory state in the body, and it is inflammation that helps kick off coronary artery disease (read pages 20-21 for more details).

In addition, I also want to make sure that you are now eating healthy all day long. To power up your diet even more, add these cholesterol-lowering foods (read pages 81-82, and 144-148 for more details).

By the end of Week 11 you should have achieved the following:

- Kept a journal as to your sleep habits. Are you getting a good night's sleep, or are you sleeping less than you realize?

- If you have symptoms of sleep apnea, make an appointment with your doctor to check it out.

- Get your teeth examined.

- Weigh yourself and chart your progress.

Week 12 — Congratulations — You're On Your Way To Victory

This week, take time to feel good about what you accomplished. If you have followed my step-by-step instructions, your kitchen should now be rid of high-fat, processed food, and, if you're following my menu plan, you probably have added some new foods to your diet that you were unfamiliar with, like tofu, perhaps. You also should be walking an hour a day, as well as doing exercises to build muscle mass. If so, I'm sure you've noticed a difference, not only in how you look, but how you feel as well. This 90-day mark is a good time to look not only at the scale, but the mirror. Your belly should be disappearing. Also, book a return visit to your doctor, and ask for lab tests to see how your target numbers have changed. If you've followed this plan, the difference should be dramatic.

By the end of Week 12 you should have achieved the following:

- You should have a journal in which you continue to track your diet, exercise and stress reduction process.

- You should be walking one hour a day and also adding in other exercise at least three times a week.

- Visit your doctor; it's time to have your target numbers checked.

Congratulate yourself — the fight is not over, but you've got the tools and you are well on your way. Keep reviewing and working on this plan, and you will be victorious and live a heart-healthy life.

CHAPTER 21

Alternative Heart Treatments

As a cardiologist, I rely on a wide variety of cardiac medications, and I also resort to the insertion of stents and coronary bypass surgery to save my patients from heart attacks. These are the mainstays for those in need of urgent intervention. But there is a role for alternative medicine as well. These treatments can be used in combination with conventional cardiac medicine to help my patients reach their target goals, or they can be used alone afterward to help them stay in optimum health.

The problem, though, is that alternative remedies are not subject to the same degree of stringent government oversight that conventional drugs and medical procedures must undergo, resulting in a maze of confusing treatments. Vast potential also exists for the marketing of ineffective, and even fraudulent treatments. So I do a lot of research before using them on my patients, and I track their results carefully.

I also warn my patients that even though an alternative remedy is labeled "natural," such as supplements distilled from herbs, they do have the power to interact with cardiac medications. This is why you should always tell your doctor about everything you take, whether it comes from the pharmacy or the health food store!

Chelation

When it comes to heart health, most of the alternative medicine area deals with supplements, but there is one popular procedure said to reduce cardiovascular disease, and this is chelation.

About 100,000 Americans undergo chelation every year, which is an intravenous process that uses EDTA, a chemical substance, to remove minerals and metals from the body that proponents believe causes heart disease. In the case of heart disease, the theory holds that these excess minerals lead to atherosclerosis, the disease process that causes coronary arteries to become narrow, leading to heart attacks.

Although I had long been skeptical of such claims, I changed my thinking after learning of the results of a large government-sponsored study. This research found that chelation, when used in conjunction with high-dose vitamins, reduced the risk of cardiovascular events by a statistically significant 26 percent.

Chelation is not cheap; it costs about $5,000 per course of treatment, and I do not recommend it in place of conventional cardiac treatment, such as drugs, and even angioplasty or bypass surgery, if needed. However, I find it a useful alternative for my patients who have heart disease that is difficult to treat medically. It can also be considered for diabetics who have small vessel coronary heart disease or foot ulcers, and for patients with other circulatory problems as well.

Supplements

Dietary supplements fall under a category that includes vitamins and minerals, along with less familiar substances like herbals, botanicals, amino acids, and enzymes. They come in a variety of forms, including tablets, capsules, softgels, gelcaps, liquids and powders. Supplements are not intended to replace a healthy diet or prescription drugs, (although they sometimes can). Supplements are intended to do exactly what their name implies — supplement for any nutritional deficiencies in your diet.

Why Take Supplements?

When I first became a cardiologist, I thought eating a wide variety of food, and perhaps add a daily multivitamin, would provide my patients with all the nutrients they needed. But I no longer think that way. Over the decades, the nutritional content of our food has changed. The word "farming" summons up a countryside image, but that isn't how things are today. Nowadays, agriculture is known as "agribusiness," with the focus on business. New farming methods speed the growing process but leach nutrients from the soil. Too many of our foods are laced with chemicals.

Multivitamins are not the total answer. They contain a selection of vitamins in amounts that meet, or exceed, the government's Recommended Daily Allowance (RDA). This is the standard amount of each vitamin or mineral that the government decrees we need to stay healthy. But many of these standards were formulated years ago and do not reflect recent (or even not that recent) research. And, even if they did, it's difficult to roll all of these nutrients into a single pill!

With this in mind, here then are alternative treatments that I have recommended to my patients along with the medical conditions that they address. Some are multifaceted and involve several products, but I've organized them according to the problems they target the most. Because of this, you'll also find them addressed in other parts of the book. But this section is designed to provide you with a more comprehensive rundown of these treatments, along with how to use them.

Overall Heart Health

CoQ10 — CoQ10 is a coenzyme, which means it's required for the enzymes in our body to function properly and, as it's found in each and every one of your body's millions of cells, it has an important role to play in the well-being of your entire body. But, in particular, this co-enzyme plays a pivotal role in heart health.

First, CoQ10 is found in the cell's mitochondria, which is the "power house" of the cell and helps produce energy, which keeps your ever-beating heart functioning properly. Unfortunately, CoQ10 production begins to lag as we age, which leads to diminished cellular energy production.

CoQ10 has additional benefits as well. It can help to lower blood pressure, and so it may help reduce the need for medication, and it also strengthens the immune system, and reduces the risk of congestive heart failure.

But there's another key reason why CoQ10 is getting attention these days. When cholesterol-lowering statin drugs were first marketed years ago, they were seen as having few side effects, but now we find that many people are developing serious muscle aches and muscle fatigue on these drugs. Taking CoQ10 can help protect against this side effect, so if you are taking statins, this coenzyme is particularly important to you. This is an additional reason why I recommend between 200 and 400 milligrams of CoQ10 daily.

Vitamin C — You may already take vitamin C when you feel a cold coming on to boost your immune system, but this vitamin does a lot more than that, especially when it comes to your heart. First, vitamin C helps reduce concentrations of C-reactive protein in the blood, which lowers heart-disease causing inflammation. It's also a powerful antioxidant. Second, vitamin C helps the coronary arteries function properly, and there is some evidence it may help lower cholesterol as well. I recommend up to 2,000 milligrams of vitamin C daily, and more if you're recovering from surgery, because it promotes healing. If your gums are receding, start taking 3,000 milligrams of vitamin C immediately, and you'll be amazed at the difference.

Vitamin D — Vitamin D, which is known as the "sunshine vitamin," is increasingly being hailed as essential to the healthy functioning of your heart, and this mirrors what I see in my own practice as well. We get vitamin D two ways: from the food we eat, and from absorbing it through our skin from sunshine. But the body's ability to synthesize vitamin D lessens as you age, so even here in Florida, many of my elderly patients are deficient, and at greater risk for high blood pressure, congestive heart failure, coronary heart disease, diabetes and even depression. If you think you are deficient in vitamin D, a blood test will show it. I look for readings in the high normal range because I find the low range of normal is unacceptable. I put my vitamin D-deficient patients on 5,000 IU for three months, after which I reduce the dosage to a 2,000 IU maintenance dose. I suggest checking the blood vitamin D level every three months until normal.

Folic Acid — Folic acid (vitamin B9) plays a crucial role in heart health because it helps produce and maintain new cells. Folic acid is also essential for the metabolism of homocysteine. This is an amino acid that is normally found in our blood, but elevated levels can damage coronary arteries. Taking folic acid helps lower homocysteine, as well as promoting normal blood platelet aggregation, which is essential to good cardiovascular health. I recommend 400 micrograms of folic acid a day for my patients whose homocysteine levels are too high.

Probiotics — The latest research shows that the bacteria that live in the gut can influence the development of heart disease. But not all types of bacteria are bad; there are helpful bacteria involved in digestion, including some that help prevent cholesterol from being reabsorbed by the body. I recommend 2-4 capsules daily.

Blood Pressure

Beet Juice — known in the UK as "beetroot juice" — is a powerful aid in reducing blood pressure. Researchers have found that drinking beet juice not only lowers blood pressure, but also delivers potent antioxidants and may help improve blood flow. But beet juice warrants some caution; taking too much can cause diarrhea. It is also a strong dye that can turn your urine and feces red. Don't worry; this is a harmless side effect. Beet juice also has an earthy taste, which some people like, but some do not. You can lessen its taste somewhat by combining it with carrot juice. If you don't care for beet juice at all, celery, lettuce, spinach, and arugula also provide nitrates.

Hawthorn — Hawthorn extract, made from the berries of the hawthorn plant, provides a number of cardiac benefits, but in particular it contains a beneficial flavonoid called proanthocyanidin, which causes the blood vessels to relax, thereby lowering blood pressure. It's available in supplement form or as a tea. I recommend one cup of tea daily.

Cholesterol Reduction

Everyone always wants to know how to lower their cholesterol without using drugs. Although these supplements do not bring your cholesterol down as effectively as statin drugs, they can be very useful either for people who cannot take statins due to side effects, or for those with mild cholesterol problems who do not need to take such powerful drugs.

Red Rice Yeast — While most supplements can't match the cholesterol-lowering effects of statin drugs, there is one that comes very close. Red rice yeast contains a substance that is chemically identical to the active ingredient in a statin drug. But quality control is a problem. Red rice yeast is manufactured in China, and there have been instances of the product being laced with a statin to enhance the effect. This is an illegal and dangerous practice.

Plant Sterols — Plant sterols, also known as plant stanols, are contained in small quantities in vegetable oils, legumes, and such grains as corn, rye and wheat, and they can be taken in supplement form as well. They are plant versions of cholesterol (our form of cholesterol is only found in humans and animals), and while you may think of cholesterol as a bad thing, it's really not. When plant sterols are consumed in sufficient amounts, they block the absorption of cholesterol in the small intestine. In fact, research finds they can lower bad cholesterol by 14 percent, similar to a statin drug. Take 2 grams a day. I prefer plant sterol supplements to products such as sterol-laced margarines and chews, because these products contain unwanted industrial ingredients.

Niacin — Niacin (vitamin B3) is a very important supplement because it lowers LDL cholesterol and triglycerides, boosts HDL cholesterol (the so-called "good" cholesterol), and transforms small, bullet-like LDL particles into a more harmless type. Start off with a low dose (250 mg) and build up to 1,500 to 3,000 mg daily. Niacin can cause flushing in 15% of individuals, so adjust the intake dosage slowly over time to prevent flushing; this may take up to one to year. Be cautious about adding niacin if you already take statins because taking both can increase the potential for adverse side effects.

Fish Oil — Throughout this book, I discuss the benefits of fish oil as a way to lower cholesterol, but I didn't want to neglect to mention it in this chapter since this supplement is viewed as part of alternative medicine. I also choose fish oil over prescription drugs as my first line of therapy to lower triglycerides, which are fats found in the blood. There is an increasing focus on triglycerides, which is now being called "the ugly cholesterol" because of its potential for increasing stroke risk even more so than the "bad" LDL cholesterol. I recommend 2,000 mg of fish oil supplement daily. If you're already taking the blood thinners Plavix or Coumadin, along with aspirin, keep an eye out for telltale bruising. This indicates that your blood is being thinned too much, and you should discontinue taking the fish oil.

Garlic — Garlic, the edible bulb of the lily plant, which is lauded for a number of beneficial cardiac effects, is also a mild cholesterol reducer. Garlic also can slightly reduce blood pressure. I recommend 1-2 capsules a day.

Flaxseed — Flaxseed, flaxseed oil and flaxseed lignans, which are concentrated in flaxseed, have a mild cholesterol-lowering effect. I tend to put some on my salads or take a spoonful a day.

Diabetes Prevention

As I point out in this book, diabetes greatly increases the risk of a heart attack. Here are some alternative treatments that can help prevent it. Remember, though, the best "alternative" way to reduce diabetes risk is to lose weight, eat heart-healthy, and exercise!

Curcumin — This is the pigment in turmeric spice that provides Indian curry its distinctive yellow color. It is also a strong anti-inflammatory that may bestow many health benefits, including helping to prevent diabetes. I suggest 2-4 capsules per day.

Chinese herbs — Chinese herbs have long been promoted for improved glucose tolerance, and there may be something to it, at least according to an Australian study. The research team at the University of Western Sydney analyzed 16 trials, which involved 1,391 people. In half of the study, those who received the Chinese herbal medications, and who modified their lifestyle, were more than twice as likely to normalize their glucose levels. But the researchers also sounded a cautious note; they observed that the participants who were the most successful also changed their lifestyle, which greatly reduces diabetes risk. In addition, they had no way to guarantee that the Chinese herbs used in each study were identical formulations.

Chromium Picolinate — Chromium picolinate is a metal that is called a "trace" mineral, because very small amounts of it are needed to maintain health. It is a multipurpose supplement which is used for various ailments including depression and polycystic ovary disease (PCOS), and is also touted as a weight loss aid. One of its major purposes, though, is in helping to prevent diabetes in people with insulin resistance, and also improving blood sugar values in people who have the disease. I recommend 200-400 mcg/day for better blood sugar control. However, I do not I recommend long-term use. To improve glucose levels, lose weight and eat foods with no or little added sugar.

Irregular Heartbeats or Palpitations

Magnesium — Magnesium is a very important mineral, and you may have heard of it in terms of its benefit in helping to strengthen bones, like vitamin D. But that's not the only role that magnesium plays in your health; this mineral also helps keep your heart beating steadily, which is particularly important if you are prone to irregular heartbeat problems. This is because it helps to suppress extra heartbeats. In addition, magnesium can play a role in helping to lower high blood pressure. I recommend taking between 300 and 600 milligrams daily.

Calcium: The Supplement You Should Not Take

Last year, a study in the journal "Heart" confirmed what I had long suspected to be true — that calcium supplements, which are targeted particularly at middle-aged women as a necessity to prevent osteoporosis, actually do little in that regard and actually cause more harm in the form of an increased risk of heart disease. So ditch the supplements and build strong bones by undertaking an exercise program of strength training three times a week and eating calcium-rich dark green vegetables.

Important Things to Consider When Choosing Supplements

Remember that supplements can be powerful agents. It's important to talk to your doctor if you are considering supplements for the following reasons:

- You take prescription drugs and you want to check about any potential interactions.

- You want to reduce or replace your need for prescription drugs.

- You are planning to have surgery, as certain supplements may increase the risk of bleeding or affect the response to anesthesia.

- In addition, follow these tips when taking supplements:

- Read the label instructions and follow them carefully. Some suggest that they be taken with food, while others note that they are suitable only for adults.

- Make a note on how many tablets must be taken each day. Some supplements claim on the label to fulfill 100 percent of your daily needs, but only if doses are taken two or three times a day (or even more).

- If you experience any health issues you think might be related to the supplement, stop taking it and contact your doctor.

- You are pregnant, are nursing a baby, or are considering giving a child a dietary supplement.

Beware Dangerous Supplements

The nation's drug supply is beset with problems due to counterfeit prescription drugs, which have flooded the market from China and other countries. But it's not only prescription drugs you need to watch out for; supplements have their problems as well. Sometimes, supplements contain dangerous ingredients, or, as in the case of prescription drugs, they may even be fakes.

Here's what to look for:

- Ask your doctor about a particular supplement you're thinking of buying.

- Look to see if the product makes mention of a manufacturer's certification on the label. Certification is not required, but there are organizations, including NSF International, a nonprofit public health and safety organization, and the Natural Products Association (NPA), an industry trade group, that offer certification to attest to manufacturing standards that are consistent with, or exceed the requirements set out by the FDA.

- Check the label to see that the nutrient you are buying is listed in the ingredients, and in what amounts. If there is wording that the amount has been "standardized," this provides added assurance.

- Choose supplements that are manufactured in the U.S. or Canada.

- Watch out for supplements sold by email or promoted in a foreign language.

- Watch out for outrageous "too good to be true" claims.

- Do your research. The National Center for Complementary and Alternative Medicine (NCCAM) and the National Institutes of Health (NIH) Office of Dietary Supplements (ODS), as well as other federal agencies, maintain information on their websites about supplements.

The Simple Heart Cure Food List

These are the main foods that comprise my Simple Heart Cure Eating Plan. These foods are part of a plant-based diet that will make your cholesterol levels plummet and help you lose weight fast, and result in normalizing your blood pressure and blood sugar levels as well. This is a list of food choices that may be familiar from other popular vegetarian or plant-based eating plans because, basically, eating this way works!

Vegetables

This list includes all green leafy vegetables, green beans, asparagus, carrots, mushrooms, Swiss chard, tomatoes. Basically, if it's a vegetable, I encourage you to eat it. The only exceptions are avocados and olives, which are high in fat. Tomato sauce and tomato paste are also allowed but, again, make sure to read the ingredients to make sure that no sugar or oil has been added.

Fruits

As with vegetables, my Simple Heart Cure Eating Plan includes all fruits, including apples, banana, blueberries, cherries, cranberries, and so on, all the way to watermelons. For the sake of variety, I also include some unusual fruits, like litchi nuts, although these must be fresh, not canned. In addition, I also allow some dried fruits, as long as they are not processed with added sugar. These include cherries, cranberries, dates, mango, papaya and raisins. Of all of these fruits, the ones that I recommend most are the berries, because of their high antioxidant levels. Fruits like apples and pears are very satisfying, and you can eat them with the skin on for added fiber. Frozen fruits are fine as well; in fact, frozen blueberries or mango chunks, eaten almost straight from the freezer, make for a refreshing treat and dessert. Make sure to choose organic!

Grains and Cereals

Bread, bagels, English muffins, crackers, etc., must be 100 percent whole wheat or whole grain, with no sugar added. Again, you have to carefully read the labels. Other grains allowed include barley, brown rice, wild rice, buckwheat, bulger, corn, corn tortillas, faro, hominy grits, kasha, millet, oatmeal, and oats. Whole-grain couscous is also a good choice. Quinoa, a grain that soaks up flavor, has become increasingly popular, and you can also eat products made with rye or spelt, and wheat tortillas.

When it comes to cereals, oatmeal, which is a combination of soluble and insoluble fiber, is an excellent cholesterol fighter. Other good cereal types that are low in calories and high in fiber include Grape-Nuts, Raisin Bran, or multigrain flakes (both without sugar), shredded wheat, Wheatena, and Uncle Sam cereal. Again, make sure to read labels and make sure that what you're buying is made from 100 percent whole grain, with no added sugar or malt.

Legumes

These vegetables include beans, peas, and lentils, and are among the most versatile and nutritious foods available. They are typically low in fat, contain low cholesterol, and are high in nutrients. They also are a good source of protein, and they are packed with soluble and insoluble fiber. In fact, they are one of the super foods that help to lower cholesterol. Legumes include all types of beans, including black-eyed peas, chick peas, lima beans, navy beans, kidney beans and more. Legumes can be your best friends when it comes to lowering your cholesterol levels, and I find many ways to include them frequently in my diet.

Protein

As an American accustomed to eating a conventional Western style diet, you are no doubt convinced that you must get your protein from red meat, poultry, or fish. This is a key reason why we have such high rates of heart disease. People in many other countries get their protein from other sources, yet they are not protein deficient. While you are getting your numbers down to your target level, it is important that you get your protein from these other sources. Legumes, as I just mentioned, are an important source of protein. The main part of my Simple Heart Cure Plan gets its protein from omega-3 egg whites, soy, and soy alternatives such as edamame, soy fat-free sausages, soy hot dogs, and tempeh, tofu, and oil-free veggie burgers.

Dairy and Dairy Substitutes
Dairy products can be another hidden source of fat that keeps your cholesterol levels sky-high. I recommend nonfat Greek yogurt, and if you do use other dairy products, like cottage cheese, sour cream, or cream cheese, make sure they are organic and nonfat. There are other types of "milk" made from other substances that are allowed, including oats, rice and soy, just make sure that they are unsweetened. Coconut water is becoming increasingly popular; just make sure it isn't flavored with sugar.

Fats and Oils
Although the whole idea of the Simple Heart Cure Eating Plan is to reduce the fats in your blood, there are some fats that you may find useful, including non-dairy salad dressing, fish oil, flaxseed oil, and nonstick cooking spray. In particular, I find olive oil cooking spray a valuable ally in the kitchen! When using any oil, only very small amounts are needed.

Herbs and Spices
Living the Simple Heart Cure lifestyle requires you to give up your salt shaker, along with processed foods, which tend to be high not only in sugar, but also sodium. But if you get to know the wonderful array of herbs and spices you have available, you won't even miss it. This list includes flavor additives like capers, chili flakes, fennel seeds, garlic, chili, green chillies, mace, mustard, natural vanilla, and pepper. Don't forget the vast array of fresh and dried herbs that are available to you. If you learn how to use herbs and spices well, your food will be bursting with both health and flavor.

Nuts
Add flavor to dishes with walnuts and almonds or snack on a small handful.

Sweeteners

Use small amounts of organic honey or pure maple syrup.

Remember:
- Choose organic foods as often as possible.
- Choose real, whole foods, and stay away from all processed foods.
- Stay away from "fake" products, like all types of margarine.
- If you use oils, use very tiny amounts.
- No artificial sweeteners or artificially sweetened products.

Dr. Crandall's Simple Heart Cure 14-Day Menu Plan

This chapter contains my 14-day Simple Heart Cure Menu Plan that will jump-start your new heart-healthy lifestyle. Personally, I enjoy eating whole fruits, vegetables, and whole grains in their fresh natural state, the way God created them. But I also know that many of my patients enjoy trying new recipes, so I've created some simple ones that you may want to try.

The recipes aren't the important part, though. What is important is that these foods are filling, and also are the most nutritious ingredients that you could ever find. They are whole foods, which means they are not processed and chemical-filled. So enjoy them.

You may also notice that elsewhere in the book there are some sections that include foods that I do not list in the Simple Heart Cure 14-Day Menu Plan, like very lean turkey or an occasional egg yolk. These are foods that you can add when you are well on your way to your victory over heart disease. But, for now, following the foods on this plan will provide you with your biggest head start. Once you've reached your target goals, you can add these other foods gradually and sparingly. Remember, though: if you do, and you find your weight, blood pressure, total cholesterol, and triglyceride levels creeping up, go back on the foods listed in this 14-day plan. Many of my patients enjoy it so much they never find any reason to change.

Tip: One of the best things about eating a plant-based diet is that you can easily mix-and-match dishes. It's important to eat a meal with a lot of protein during the day so you don't get hungry, but don't hesitate to swap out lunches for dinners. Also, if you are very hungry, just add more fruits and vegetables! When you eat this way, you can't go wrong!

Your All-Important Breakfast

If you are a breakfast skipper, or if you just grab a roll (or, even worse, a muffin or donut) as you fly out the door, you must stop this behavior right now! That also goes for a bowl of sugar coated cereal, even those that are promoted as "healthy." Such breakfasts will leave you hungry by 10 a.m. On the other hand, these hearty breakfasts provide you with the high-quality fuel your body needs to function properly.

I always recommend that my patients start the day with what I've come to call Dr. Crandall's Favorite Breakfast. Don't be surprised, though, if you end up enjoying my favorite breakfast two or three times a week, and eventually all of the time. Many of my patients do, and I do too!

One of the reasons I prefer this type of breakfast, which includes protein from eggs, is that it's protein that keeps you from getting hungry by mid-morning. If you prefer one of the oatmeal or cereal-type breakfasts listed here, and you find yourself getting hungry, add a scrambled egg white and eat it on the side.

You can end your meals with coffee or tea. Coffee can be lightened with a splash of almond milk, if you like.

WEEK ONE

Monday

Breakfast — Dr. Crandall's Scrambled Eggs and Whole Wheat Sugar Free Toast

½ cup fresh blueberries

Quick Recipe: Scramble three omega-3 egg whites in a non-stick pan that you've coated lightly with an olive oil cooking spray. Take a piece of whole wheat bread and brown it in the oven until toasted. Enjoy the whole wheat toast with sugar-free blueberries.

Lunch — Fresh Spinach Salad

Quick Recipe: Toss spinach leaves with vegetables such as sliced mushrooms, chopped carrot, chopped apple, and toss in a few raisins and walnuts as well.

2 Wasa crackers topped with nonfat, organic cream cheese

Dinner — Bountiful Roasted Vegetables

Side salad of lettuce, cucumber and cherry tomatoes, dressed with balsamic vinegar

Quick Recipe: Cut or chop an assortment of any type of vegetables you want (zucchini, onion, bell peppers and sweet potatoes are good examples) and place on a baking sheet that you've sprayed with a small amount of olive oil cooking spray. Spray a little of the cooking spray on top and bake in a 400-degree oven until the vegetables are tender.

Tofu slices in a bowl topped with cinnamon and walnuts covered with a small amount of real maple syrup.

Tuesday

Breakfast — Whole-Grain French Toast Topped with Strawberries

Tea or coffee

Quick Recipe: Soak one slice of sugar-free, whole grain bread in a bowl with three beaten omega-3 egg whites. You can add cinnamon or vanilla to the eggs if desired.

Cook bread on a non-stick pan or a pan lightly coated with olive oil cooking spray. While the mixture is cooking, pour the remaining eggs over the bread.

Top with fresh strawberries and a small amount of real maple syrup.

Lunch — Mixed Three Bean Salad

Quick Recipe: Drain and rinse canned cannelloni beans, kidney beans, and garbanzo beans. Add some chopped celery, parsley, and red onion. Toss with apple cider vinegar and a small amount of honey.

½ cup fresh pineapple topped with nonfat yogurt (you can mix in some vanilla and just a tiny bit of pure maple syrup if you'd like).

Dinner

Grilled oil-free veggie burger served on whole-wheat sugar-free bun topped with lettuce, tomato and onion slice

Sliced dill pickle

One cup steamed carrots, lightly dusted with cinnamon

Wednesday

Breakfast

1 cup of old-fashioned cooked oatmeal (never instant!) topped with a handful of raisins

½ sliced banana and a splash of sugar free almond milk if desired

Lunch — Strawberry Spinach Salad

Combine the spinach with sliced strawberries, and drizzle with a bit of balsamic vinegar and honey to sweeten.

½ cup of nonfat Greek yogurt, topped with chunks of fresh or frozen mango

Dinner — Bruschetta Topped Whole Wheat Toast

Quick Recipe: Stir together chopped ripe plum tomatoes, a few chopped fresh basil leaves, a chopped garlic clove, and some olive oil to moisten the mix (but as sparingly as possible). Spoon the mixture on to just toasted whole-wheat sugar-free bread and slice into squares. Put the mixture on top just before serving so it doesn't get soggy.

½ cup nonfat cottage cheese topped with fresh or frozen peaches

Thursday

Breakfast — Mexican-Style Omelet

Quick Recipe: Brown chopped onions and peppers in a pan lightly sprayed with olive oil cooking spray. Scramble three omega-3 egg whites and add a pinch of cumin, a pinch of garlic powder and a pinch of chopped cilantro. Serve folded in an organic, sugar-free corn tortilla.

½ cup fresh blueberries

Lunch — Quinoa Black Bean Salad

Quick Recipe: Make quinoa according to the packaged instructions. In a bowl, combine one-teaspoon olive oil, a squeeze of fresh lime juice, pinch of cumin, coriander, fresh cilantro, minced scallions, diced tomatoes, and cut up bell pepper. Stir in drained, canned black beans. Mix with the cooled quinoa.

Dinner — Greek Tofu Salad

Quick Recipe: Cut firm tofu into chunks the size of dice and press it with paper towels to absorb any water. Steam the tofu for five minutes. Whisk together a small amount of olive oil, wine vinegar, basal, black pepper, oregano, and salt. Pour this mixture over the tofu and let it marinate. Meanwhile, chop up some fresh tomato, cucumber, and red onions and toss together with the chunks of tofu.

Dessert: Top ½ cup low-fat yogurt with chopped dates and raisins and dust with cinnamon

Friday

Breakfast

1 cup shredded wheat (no sugar). Serve with one sliced banana and non-sweetened almond milk.

Tea or coffee

Lunch — Cold Green Bean Salad with Basil and Tomatoes

Quick Recipe: Quickly cook whole string beans lightly so they are still crunchy, not limp. Drain and refrigerate until cold. Lightly sprinkle them with a bit of olive oil and red wine vinegar and serve the beans over large slices of ripe tomato. Top with fresh basil leaves.

½ cup fresh cantaloupe

Dinner — Baked Potato Topped with Nonfat Organic Sour Cream (or Nonfat Greek Yogurt) and Chives

1 cup roasted brussels sprouts with balsamic vinegar

Quick Recipe: Slice fresh brussels sprouts in half, place them in a single layer on a baking pan sprayed with olive oil spray, and drizzle the balsamic vinegar over them and make sure they are coated. Bake for 20 minutes in a 375 degree oven.

Saturday

Breakfast — Scrambled Omega-3 Eggs with Baked Home Fries

½ cup fresh mango chunks

1 slice whole-wheat sugar-free toast

Quick Recipe: Cut up small potatoes, spread them on a cooking sheet that you've coated with a small amount of olive oil cooking spray, arrange them on the cooking sheet, and lightly spray them again with cooking spray. Dust with pepper if you wish. Bake in a preheated 475 degree oven for 15-20 minutes, or until tender but crispy.

Lunch — Nonfat Cottage Cheese with Cut-Up Cucumbers and Tomatoes

1 slice sugar-free whole-wheat bread spread with nonfat herb and garlic cream cheese

1 cup steamed broccoli tossed with minced garlic and a squeeze of lemon juice

Dinner — Portobello Basil Sandwich

Quick Recipe: Stir lemon juice and nonfat yogurt into a bowl, and brush over the sides of a large 4-ounce mushroom cap (stem removed, caps sliced). Grill or broil the mushroom until tender (2-3 minutes). Toast two slices of whole-wheat sugar-free bread under the broiler. Spread half of the lemon juice/nonfat yogurt mixture on the toasted bread and arrange fresh basil leafs and sliced tomatoes on top. Cut and serve.

Sunday

Breakfast — Banana Omelet

½ cup Fresh strawberries

Tea or coffee

Quick Recipe: Scramble three omega-3 egg whites and pour in an olive oil spray-treated pan and cook as you would an omelet. Before you flip it, cover with banana slices. Top with cinnamon.

Lunch — Watermelon Salad
Quick Recipe: ½ cup watermelon, balled or cut into chunks, ½ cup fresh mint leaves, baby greens. Arrange the watermelon on the plate, and top with the fresh mint leaves and the baby greens.

2 Wasa crackers topped with nonfat cream cheese and dusted with cinnamon

Dinner — Grilled Tofu Salad with Veggies
Quick Recipe: Grill the tofu and slice. Place 1 cup of arugula, 1 tbsp. balsamic vinegar, ½ cup of chopped onions, one quartered red tomato, ½ cup raw carrots, and 1 cut up small cucumber in a bowl. Top with slices of grilled tofu and drizzle with balsamic vinegar.

Snacks
On my Simple Heart Cure Menu Plan, you can have snacks. Enjoy fruits and vegetables in their fresh, natural state or, if you prefer, jazz them up. Here are some ideas to get you started:

- Orange with mint. Peel and cut up an orange and combine with chopped mint

- Two dates with a cup of tea

- A small glass of low alcohol content red wine or organic grape juice, two Wasa crackers and a handful of grapes

- pple slices dusted with cinnamon

- ½ cup nonfat Greek yogurt with fresh raspberries stirred in

- Celery sticks stuffed with organic nonfat organic cottage cheese and chopped chives

- Two Wasa crackers topped with nonfat organic cream cheese

- Two dates stuffed with softened nonfat cream cheese

- Tofu slices in a bowl topped with cinnamon and walnuts covered with a small amount of real maple syrup. (This is my favorite dessert, and it also makes a great snack!)

WEEK TWO

Monday

Breakfast — Scrambled Eggs and Cottage Cheese Omelet

Quick Recipe: Pour three beaten omega-3 egg whites in a non-stick pan that you've coated lightly with olive oil cooking spray. When the eggs begin to thicken slightly, spoon in one or two tablespoons of nonfat organic cottage cheese. Flip over omelet style, dust with cinnamon and serve.

½ cup fresh berries (any type)

Lunch — Sicilian Salad

Quick Recipe: Peel and slice one large navel orange and arrange on plate, alternating with slices of red onion. Sprinkle with basil leaves and walnuts and drizzle with a tiny amount of balsamic vinegar. Sprinkle with pepper.

1 slice no sugar whole-wheat toast

½ cup blueberries

Dinner — Black Beans and Brown Rice

Quick Recipe: Cook the brown rice and heat a can of drained black beans. Chop up some onion, red, yellow, or green peppers, chopped cilantro, a teaspoon ground cumin and a pinch of cayenne pepper. Cook the chopped vegetables, add the spices and add the beans. Spoon it over the rice.

Chunks of melon with sliced strawberries

Tuesday

Breakfast

1 cup nonfat cottage cheese served with one cup of fresh berries (any type or mix of berries, such as blueberries, raspberries, strawberries and blackberries)

1 slice sugar-free whole-wheat toast

Lunch — Rainbow Fruit Salad

Quick Recipe: Blend one cup of nonfat Greek yogurt with ½ ripe banana and a squeeze of lemon juice. Cut up a papaya, a mango, and a pear. Pour the yogurt dressing over the fruit.

2 Wasa crackers

Dinner — Roasted Beets and Sweet Potatoes

Quick Recipe: Cut beets and sweet potatoes into one-inch cubes. Arrange them on a baking pan wrapped in tin foil and coated with cooking spray, then also spray them on top with cooking spray. Bake until tender (about 35 minutes).

½ cup nonfat Greek yogurt with blueberries and strawberries mixed in

Wednesday

Breakfast — Veggie Scrambled Eggs

Beat three omega-3 egg whites. Add an assortment of chopped vegetables, such as spinach, green and red peppers, mushrooms, and onions — whatever veggies are on hand. Scramble and serve.

1 slice whole-wheat sugar-free bread, toasted

½ cup fresh cherries

Lunch — Oil-free Veggie Burger Topped with Oven-Roasted Peppers

Small green salad of spinach, lettuce, cucumber and tomato, dressed with red wine or balsamic vinegar

Quick Recipe: Place a whole red or green pepper on a baking sheet and broil until the skin has turned black and blistery. Remove from the oven and place the peppers into an airtight container, like a paper or plastic bag or covered bowl. Wait 10-15 minutes, then remove and slide off the skin. Cut the pepper in half, remove the core and seeds, and slice into strips to top your burger.

Dinner — Veggie Stuffed Sweet Potato
Quick Recipe: Bake one sweet potato, then cut off the top and scoop out the inside without breaking the skin. Mash the inside of the potato in a bowl. Stir in thawed frozen organic peas, corn, beans, and carrots — any small vegetable pieces you like. Restuff the potato skin and return to the oven for 15 minutes to brown.

½ cup fat free Greek yogurt with raspberries and sliced banana

Thursday

Breakfast — Whole Grain French Toast with Blueberry Compote
Quick Recipe: Prepare the whole grain French toast according to the directions in Week One. Place in 1 cup fresh blueberries, 1 tsp. vanilla extract and cook in a pan gently over low heat for 15 minutes.

Lunch — Lentil Salad
Take 1 cup of chilled, steamed lentils and toss with chopped red peppers, cubed cucumber, and diced red onions. Toss with balsamic vinegar and dust with pepper if desired.

2 Wasa Crackers

Dinner — Whole Wheat Pasta Primavera
Quick Recipe: Prepare pasta according to package instructions. Heat a nonstick skillet and add a little water to prevent sticking when you sauté. Sauté some diced bell pepper, onion, garlic cloves, tomatoes, and scallions. Add to the just cooked pasta, stir, and serve.

Friday

Breakfast — Scrambled Eggs with Browned Onions and Peppers
Quick recipe: Beat three omega-3 egg whites in a bowl and set aside. Spray a non-stick skillet with a small amount of olive oil spray and heat it until it's hot, then add chopped onions. Cook until the onions are brown, stirring constantly to prevent burning, until they are caramelized. Add some diced green peppers and cook until tender, then pour on the egg whites and scramble in the pan.

Whole-Wheat English muffin (sugar-free)

Lunch — Indian Cucumber and Yogurt Salad

Quick Recipe: Peel and remove the seeds from one cucumber and slice thin. Mix with one clove chopped garlic. Pour off any liquid that has formed and mix in 1 tablespoon dried mint. Beat nonfat plain yogurt until smooth, pour over cucumber mixture and refrigerate. Serve over lettuce.

Veggie Burger with Oven-Baked "French Fries"

Quick Recipe: Slice one potato into strips. Arrange on baking sheet coated with a very small amount of olive oil cooking spray. Spray the potato strips with the cooking spray. Bake at 450 degrees for 30 minutes or until golden. Sprinkle with pepper if desired.

Dinner — Roasted Eggplant with Lemon

Easy Recipe: Coat a baking pan with cooking spray. Take an eggplant that you've sliced in half and quartered, and place on the baking sheet, skin side down. Spray with a small amount of cooking spray. Roast in the oven at 400 degrees until softened and brown. Remove from the oven and sprinkle with lemon juice.

Steamed baby carrots dusted with cinnamon

One 6-ounce glass of low alcohol red wine or organic grape juice

Saturday

Breakfast — Apple Cinnamon Oatmeal

In a small pot, add ¼ cup of water, ½ chopped apple, a small handful of raisins, a tsp. of vanilla, and cinnamon and simmer until the apple is soft. Cook your oatmeal as usual and combine with the fruit mixture. Add a splash of almond milk if desired.

Lunch — Quinoa Salad with Dried Fruits

Cook quinoa until it is tender. Add some chopped celery, chopped green onions, raisins, dried cranberries, a splash of distilled white vinegar, a splash of lemon juice, and a pinch of cayenne pepper; mix together. Stand at room temperature before serving.

Dinner — Whole Wheat Penne with Broccoli

Quick Recipe: Prepare the penne according to the package directions. Cut 1 bunch of broccoli into florets, and, when 3 minutes of cooking time remain for the pasta, add the broccoli. Remove from the heat, drain pasta and broccoli and return to pot, stir in some fresh halved cherry tomatoes and fresh basil leaves and serve.

One 6-oz glass low alcohol content red wine or a small glass of organic grape juice.

Sunday

Breakfast — Breakfast Burrito

Quick Recipe: Coat a nonstick pan with olive oil cooking spray. Mix three omega-3 egg whites (or the equivalent) into a bowl, and add 1 tbsp. chopped raw scallions, 1 tbsp. raw cilantro and ½ cup of black beans. Scramble the egg mixture and then fold into a whole-wheat tortilla. Top with fresh chopped tomatoes and cilantro.

Lunch — Tomato Salad with Fresh Greens

Quick Recipe: Take 1 cup of fresh mesclun greens and toss with two tablespoons red wine vinegar. Arrange the greens over sliced fresh tomatoes. Drizzle with a chive dressing made from fresh chopped chives mixed into non-fat yogurt.

½ cup of nonfat cottage cheese with fresh peaches

Dinner — Garden Fresh Cottage Cheese Salad with Whole Wheat Penne

Quick Recipe: To nonfat cottage cheese, add chopped plum tomatoes, scallions, onions, and chopped peppers to taste, and sprinkle with pepper if desired. Serve with whole wheat penne.

Baked Apple

Hollow out one apple and squeeze a little lemon juice on the inside to prevent burning. Bake in a 400-degree oven for about 20 minutes. Sprinkle with cinnamon.

The Simple Heart Cure Shopping List

In this shopping list, you'll find ingredients for the two-week Simple Heart Cure Eating Plan listed in the book. Many of the ingredients, like the herbs and spices, you already have on hand. If you want to try all of the suggested recipes, these are the ingredients they contain. Remember, choose organic foods whenever possible, and always use real foods—nothing artificial or fake!

WEEK ONE

Almond milk (unsweetened)

Apples

Baby carrots

Balsamic vinegar

Banana

Basil (fresh)

Bell peppers

Blueberries (fresh or frozen is fine)

Black pepper

Broccoli

Brussels sprouts

Cannelloni beans

Cantaloupe

Carrots

Celery

Cherry tomatoes

Cilantro

Cinnamon

Cucumber

Cumin

Dates

Dill pickle

Dried mint

Eggplant

Garbanzo beans

Garlic

Grape juice (organic)

Kidney beans

Lemon (for juice)

Lettuce

Mango (fresh or frozen)

Mint leaves (fresh)

Mushrooms

Nonfat Greek yogurt

Nonfat cream cheese

Nonfat herb and chive cream
cheese

Oatmeal (old-fashioned type,
not instant)

Olive oil cooking spray

Omega-3 eggs

Onion

Quinoa

Plum tomatoes

Portabella mushroom

Potato

Raisins

Red wine (low alcohol content)

Red onion

Red wine vinegar

Shredded wheat (no sugar)

Scallions

Spinach

Strawberries

String beans (whole)

Sweet potato

Tofu

Tomatoes

Veggie burger (oil-free)

Walnuts

Watermelon

Whole-wheat sugar-free bread

Wine vinegar

Wasa crackers

WEEK TWO

Almond milk (unsweetened)

Balsamic vinegar

Blueberries

Banana

Basil (fresh)

Bell pepper

Black beans

Black pepper

Blueberries

Broccoli

Brown rice

Cayenne pepper

Celery

Cilantro

Cinnamon

Cucumber

Cumin

Dried cranberries

Frozen vegetables (organic
peas, corn, beans or carrots)

Garlic

Green onions (also known as
scallions)

Honeydew melon

Lemon (for juice)

Lentils

Mango

Mesclun greens

Oatmeal (old-fashioned type,
not instant)

Omega-3 eggs

Olive oil cooking spray

Navel orange
Nonfat cottage cheese
Nonfat Greek yogurt
Papaya
Pear
Peaches
Plum tomatoes
Raspberries
Red onion
Scallions
Strawberries
Sweet potatoes
Tomatoes
Vanilla extract
Veggie burger (oil-free)
Walnuts
Whole-wheat no sugar English
   muffin
Whole-wheat pasta
Whole-wheat penne pasta
Whole-wheat sugar-free bread

CONCLUSION

I wish I could say that there's a silver bullet that will cure heart disease, but there just isn't.

Heart disease is often described as a "lifestyle disease" because a life with little exercise and a diet high in fat and sugar contribute to the buildup of plaque in the arteries. Simply put, those are the causes of heart disease.

Yet, we all know people who live to a ripe old age eating fried food and doing little more exercise than puttering around the house. Meanwhile, others die in their 30s from massive coronaries. What makes the difference in their health?

Chronic stress plays a major role, as do genetics and inflammatory conditions resulting from viruses and infections. Hormonal imbalances, thyroid conditions, over-production of insulin, and many more factors can also trigger heart disease. These triggers help bring on "cardiac events" — including heart attacks, embolisms, aneurysms, and stroke.

With every new patient, I want to learn everything I can about their symptoms and history; treat the disease so I can stop it in its tracks; and then reverse it so they can lead a long and happy life because I have a profound belief that God has given everyone a role to play on this Earth.

As a committed Christian, I have found that people of faith often are more prepared than others to follow their path to true wellness. They typically have more self-discipline as a result of their powerful belief in having something to live for — a purpose larger than themselves.

So I talk and even pray with my patients about their relationship with God. I treat hearts. But we have souls, too, and both must be healthy in order to live a full life.

I've found that spiritual disciplines, such as prayer and fasting have aided my patients in their recoveries and enriched their lives.

When I first began practicing cardiology, I saw heart-attack patient after heart-attack patient come through the doors. We could help stabilize these patients and prescribe a few drugs, but there wasn't much else we could do. Many people in that era had multiple heart attacks; if they didn't die from the first one they were often left debilitated.

That's just not true anymore. We have learned so much and are learning more every day. New therapies not only are on the horizon but also are being used today. The best of medicine — from conventional medicine to alternative therapies — can help you get well. It's really true!

You have to do your part, too, of course. A doctor often will remind a patient of that fact as the patient leaves the office. The patient usually nods and makes promises. But both doubt that it's actually going to happen, and with good reason.

Habits are hard to change, and many of the habits that contribute to heart disease have been developed throughout a person's life. These habits often are associated, as well, with the best things in life — such as sitting with the family around a table that's groaning with "comfort food."

The philosopher Aristotle believed that virtue is a habit. Unfortunately, vice is a habit, too, and those unhealthy habits contribute to heart disease. Making the transition from a lifetime of bad habits to good ones is a gradual process. Coaching is important. It's the key to your success.

That's why I'm not content with simply prescribing a course of treatment for my patients, hearing their promises, and sending them on their way. I want to see them in my office on a regular basis. Their progress should be monitored, and they need to be encouraged and to remain accountable.

Patients must reeducate themselves and retool to learn to live a healthier life.

Changing habits is undoubtedly the most important part of any recovery process.

That's why I'm so glad you read this book. Consider it a "virtual visit" with one of your doctors. (It should not, however, be considered a substitute for consulting with your personal physician. I would never advise that.)

I believe strongly that, having read this book, you will concentrate on the changes you need to make. You'll be able to take advantage of the latest therapies that can make the battle easier. You'll be assured that you are up-to-date in the reeducation and retooling process.

Most of all, you'll know that you've taken the first step in the battle to ensure your better heart health. My team and I will be praying for your complete victory!

Chauncey Crandall, M.D.

Get your free online heart health assessment at
www.simpleheart411.com.

INDEX

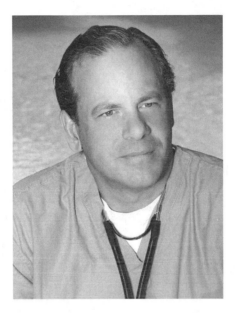

Chauncey Crandall, M.D.

Chauncey W. Crandall IV, M.D., F.A.C.C., is Director of Preventive Medicine at the renowned Palm Beach Cardiovascular Clinic and Chief of Interventional Cardiology at Good Samaritan Medical Center in Palm Beach, Florida. He is also the editor of the popular medical newsletter, Dr. Crandall's Heart Health Report.

Dr. Crandall received his post-graduate training at Yale University School of Medicine, where he also completed three years of research in the Cardiovascular Surgery Division.

In his over 25-year career, Dr. Crandall has performed over 40,000 heart procedures. He regularly lectures nationally and internationally on preventive cardiology, cardiology healthcare of the elderly, healing, interventional cardiology, and heart transplantation.

Dr. Crandall has been heralded for his values and message of hope to all his heart patients.